Chainmale
3SM

Chainmale
3SM

A Unique View of Leather Culture

Don Bastian

Published by **Daedalus Publishing Company**, 2140 Hyperion Ave., Los Angeles, CA 90027 USA

Edited by
Kari Svendsboe
and
A. Handful

Cover design by
Kari Svendsboe

Illustration by
Don Bastian

ISBN 1-881943-15-1

Printed in the United States of America

For Ron and Matt
my 'boys'

Author's Note:

If you have opened the cover of this manuscript, then you either have a general interest in what I perceive the 'gay-male-leather-scene' to be (from my somewhat limited exposure) or, I have cornered and coerced you into reading it.

Of the many people who have contributed to my education in this lifestyle that I have come to embrace, Guy Baldwin and Joseph Bean have had the most impact, and I want to take this opportunity to thank them. I may not have always agreed with their views, but I have tremendous respect for their abilities to communicate a wealth of knowledge to this 'country boy' growing up in the 'last teepee from the campfire'.

There are many people mentioned in these pages, some will recognize themselves in the events described, others will read with vague familiarity those things that happen to all of us. To them, I extend my thanks for they have shared in a world that I believe to be one of the more passionate, caring, and honest environments ever encountered.

The name for this project originated because of several viewpoints. One being the thought that our 'leathers' are to some degree a visual 'armor', a rough take-off on the Chainmail. Also, that the Leather culture, as seen from my eyes, is the result of generational education, or each experience becoming a link in the chain of self-awareness as a community and a culture. And lastly, men in Bondage; whether mentally imprisoned in the worlds of denial and fear, or actually acting out fantasies of domination, and submission.

3SM is a convenient play on words reflecting my relationship in a loving, Leather, three-way relationship: a threesome.

Introduction:

The thoughts on these pages are personal interpretations of a very complex, diverse, and rich culture. And although nothing is meant to be judgemental, the views I share are just that; my views at the time of this writing. Doubtless, as I mature in this community, some of those views may evolve with time and new explorations.

SM
Sensuality and **M**utuality
Sensory **M**agnification
Sex **M**agic
Stage **M**anagement
Stand and **M**odel
Sit and **M**oan
Sado**m**asochism
I have even heard it called **S**illy and **M**ake-believe, or **S**ick and
Maladjusted. It depends on your point of view I guess or, on whether or
not you are on your knees at the time.

Crack! *   **Delicious, that sound.***

Strange how that sound, even without knowing it's source, stirs some primal urge, feeds some deep need.

Concentrate now. That eternity before the whip splits the air, traveling so fast that it breaks the sound barrier, feeling that energy build from my shoulder to my arm, traveling down the length of the whip and feeding both our needs.

Crack!   ***Empowering. Escape. Release. Hunger.***

Always that temporary release from hunger, but never for very long because the hunger always returns...

Crack!

I love to watch the crimson tracks rise off their barren backs. I love to read their responses, and watch the tissue talk to me. Not with the grunts or gasps that escape through the vocal cords, but with the silent ripples of language that the body can only pro- duce under such extreme hunger, such communicative need, such love.

Yes, love. Reciprocal. Nurturing. How easy it is to give of your love; to care enough to give someone your innermost feelings and your heart. But have you ever cared enough for someone to give them your pain? Shared your vulnerabilities and insecu- rities to the point of such openness, not locked away or hidden like a nagging doubt, but face to face with the need to lay your self open and share the tolerance levels, that threshold just beneath the surface of such pain? Let someone empower you with the knowledge that you can explore all the parameters of your desires, wants, and needs without judgment, and trusted to the point of pain?

Crack!

Cleansing; that kind of trust. Honesty. Knowing that at any time you can signal to stop and all that euphoria will slowly recede into a physical numbness, and eventually a loneliness, and you can no longer fight off the pangs of hunger returning until that

11

dark curtain of doubt is once again rent from you back.

Crack!

I drop the whip into my left hand and slowly reach out to caress his back. Gently, barely touching it, I trace the outlines. He shivers from the warmth of my hand, the electricity our bodies share, and the reassurance my touch offers.

"Yes. I am here and you are safe with me. Relax and flow with the pain.

At what intensity it is delivered or received is irrelevant. The knowledge that it is shared is enough.

"Relax. Breathe," I whisper.

My arms encircle him and he moans. I can feel his heart beat through his rib cage as he leans back against my chest. He rocks his head back into my shoulder and I hear his breathing subside as I lay my ear against his sweaty neck. I release my arms from his chest, loosen the wrist restraints, and stroke the blood back into his arms.

"That was..."

I cut him off.

"Quiet now! Just relax. Settle down on the floor and just rest in my arms. "

It wasn't long before he dozed in that safe euphoric sleep that follows such wild, emotional explorations. I gently laid him on the floor, gathered a blanket from under the cabinet in the corner, and covered his lithe naked body.

I am always amazed at how easily the young men I share an experience with reach that safe emptiness that allows such a deep, satisfying sleep.

I recall the struggle I had. The turmoil and the difficulty reaching that state of consciousness that would allow me to let go and float in the depths of my own soul. The mentor I had chosen would never show his frustration, but I could feel that telepathic disappointment whenever I pulled back, not

12

trusting myself enough to really let go.

He was beyond patient. We rarely talked, but in five years, he guided me through a lifetime of his experience; teaching, correcting, and passing along all that he knew... a wisdom that I am just now beginning to grasp - one that parallels the world of black leather that we choose to inhabit.

I was so unlike that young man. That 'boy' that had laid at my feet before me. I came from a world that did not have such immediate media revelations. Unavailable to me were the books, videos, and magazines on the 'how-to's' of a world that only existed in our imaginations, or maybe some far off place that I may never get to experience like San Francisco, or New York. Sure, we all heard the rumors of the magical places like the Catacombs, or the Mineshaft, but their existence only fueled my imagination, and ignited thoughts of lust on those lonely, inescapable nights.

Hard to believe it had all come down to this... my sanctuary... my alter... my playroom. Many men had tested their 'right of passage' into this room. I glance around my most familiar personal space. A black, ominous jail cell is built into the brick and I can come and go when they are blindfolded. Built into the same wall is a set of stocks, lovingly carved out of fir by one of my boys. They are framed with heavy upright beams and several heights of eye-bolts decorate the sides.

Behind me, a sling is suspended from a gridwork of hooks strategically mounted in the ceiling for maneuverability and very adaptable use. On my left is a toy wall. A plethora of instruments of pleasure/torture, depending on your view, I suppose. The row of whips must be quite intimidating to a first time viewer. And the butt plugs and dildos are placed at a very convenient height to accommodate a short reach from the sling.

I smile with satisfaction as I take a deep breath, inhaling the scent of leather and enjoying the familiarity at a glance. Nothing is out of place. Everything is kept clean and orderly as befitting this room. Almost reverent... definitely spiritual... this space.

Crack!

My gaze returns to the boy on the floor as he stirs. This is what it is all about. Spirituality. The personal sacrifice, sharing and bonding. I feel the power of the 'scene' coursing thought my veins; the strength of the 'gift' that we both share, satisfying our needs. The depth of his 'want' answering the primal hunger at the end of my whip.

I become more aware of the warmth of the room as sweat trickles down my spine into my leather pants. The smell of wax permeates the air and the slow thump of the music fades during our 'dark dance' of passion.

"Thank you Sir," murmurs the boy as he curls up under a blanket in a fetal position resting his cheek on my boot.

I nudge him lightly, pulling my foot out from under him.

"That was very well done, boy," I said, as I knelt next to him, stroking his hair.

"Sir," was all he said in response. He flipped the blanket aside to reveal an erection.

"Sir?" he asked again, not daring to look up. He would never match my gaze eye to eye. He knew he had to wait for my permission.

"Go ahead, I would like to watch."

Immediately, his eyes close and he whimpers softly as his fist forms around his cock.

I usually find sex anti-climactic after a good scene, and had learned long ago not to spoil the mood with it. But I also knew what a reward this was to the boy, so I indulged myself with the view.

I have been exploring my world of Leather for over ten years now, and I am still no closer to being able to define the 'needs' I have grown to accept. Glimpses of visions that reflect what? Past lives? Maybe. Perhaps future revelations. Who knows. Almost like a camera on slow shutter-speed, my mind clicks open to a view that is not quite comprehensible, yet definitely there, clear and too real. Just glimpses, nothing to grasp coherently, but extremely satisfying at the same time. Almost reassuring. Madness.

Split personalities? No. Just an awareness that parallels my 'needs'. I came into this world of Leather quite by accident. In those days, no one advertised their interest. At least I didn't think so. In retrospect, I am not so sure I wasn't just missing the signals. They were discreet.

I fell in love with a man, also quite by accident. It was all there. The passion, the magic and the sex. Wild and free, awakening something I had not felt before. Releasing an abandonment of my worldly cares. Of course, I didn't know that then. Only looking back can I see the changes that happened.

Then, quite out of the blue, in this new-found freedom of charged sexuality, something happened. Just a word, or phrase, nothing blatant or overt. I don't think he even realized the shift in approach, the clues were so small. But when the awareness sunk in that we were 'role-playing', our sex became even more charged, more electric, and we were able to define our roles as satisfying mutual needs. Of course, it wasn't this clinically clear at the time, just extremely hot and fun. Up to this point, we had not even discussed role-play. Body language and spontaneous reactions fed our infant feelings. But it all came crashing down with the first verbal acknowledgment of the expectations.

"Call me Sir!"

There it was. Right out in the open.

"I said, call me Sir, boy."

My whole fantasy world was shattered when he uttered those words. Such vehemence was intoned. I felt belittled, worthless, and excited. Yes - excited. Yet, terrified of giving in or of giving up; giving up what I didn't know. That period of adjustment, with my own fears flooding to the surface, required a lot of talk between us.

We didn't have all the catch phrases or guidance from a known peer group to rely on. Phrases like safe, sane and consensual, or safe words that allowed an escape route emotionally from the scene. We didn't even know anyone else who 'played', other than the characters in some one-handed paperback novel.

We know things happened in the larger centers where anonymous people gathered in subterranean pleasure palaces acting out their fantasies. But to come to the realization that we were face to face with our own visceral needs, so far away from a climate of understanding, was somewhat frightening.

Little did I know that the couple next door probably did the same things we did, with or without some of the 'toys' to enhance the environment. It just somehow seemed that I had to deal with acceptance all over again. To be out and gay was one thing, but to be out and gay in a Leather sense seemed a double blow.

I always knew I was different, but was I different to the point of being a threat to my own sanity? Help came, as it always does, from within. I don't even remember the circumstances except that there were a lot of people around - a picnic or party or gathering of some kind. The conversation was about ghosts or spirits or some related topic. People were discussing, with quite open frankness, having witnessed certain phenomena and I talked about having seen what I thought was a ghost or vision when I used to tend a garden at a cemetery during my high school summer vacations.

Pretty brave stuff, to tell a group that you have seen a ghost. But no one laughed or was condescending in any way. They accepted it. I remember being almost embarrassed that no one challenged me. I also remember having the revelation that I could express my view without the threat of scorn.

Around the same time and quite by accident, I came across *The Leatherman's Handbook* written by Larry Townsend. This had been floating around circles of those-in-the-know for a few years by this time, but for me it was the first tangible evidence that the world of sadomasochism had a history applied to the gay culture. I slowly began to associate the things that had happened in my childhood, and even my recent past, with the life I was fearfully drawn to now.

I remember standing on the ranch house verandah where I grew up, watching the hired hand ride up on his horse. The smell of dust and horse sweat permeated the air, and as he pulled off his gloves, I could smell the leather sweat on his hands. He would reach out for me, and pull me close, then throw me in the air above his head. I was just four years old then, and the hired hand was my uncle. I loved him. I loved how masculine he was, how rugged, yet gentle and caring.

I look back on his life now and recall the stacks of Western Horseman and Real West magazines he used to collect, almost as if he was part of some forgotten wild frontier. He never married and died a lonely, bitter man when I was in my twenties. I often wondered if he had been searching for the strong masculine company of another man in the pages of those magazines.

Although I had proven my manhood in sports as a teenager, either by mountain climbing, wind surfing, or diving, I never managed to outrun that

16

image of my uncle. Silent. Strong. Powerful stuff, those childhood memories. Maybe because of my uncle, I always had this attraction to the loners and rebels in movies. Through puberty and my teenage years, I was always attracted to the super-masculine types. They were usually the over-characterized 'bad-guys' such as Marlon Brando and Peter Fonda in those terrible 'B' biker movies. Not until much later in life did I start to associate that all these things shaped where I am at this moment.

Horses. Bikers. Leather. All that painful hard work on the ranch. A place that I hated with a vengeance for it's loneliness. Never could I have dreamed that there existed places of crowded masculinity that I would come to love in Leather bars. Yet now, as much as I enjoy social spaces, I also have come to enjoy my time alone. Everything comes full circle.

Crack!

I am drawn out of my thoughts by the gasps of orgasm racking the boy at my feet. He discharges all over the carpet and my boots. He has had his reward, now I will have mine.

"You made a mess on my boots, boy, now lick it off, and you better make damn sure they shine!"

"Yes, Sir," he replied, a little too eagerly. And, as I smeared his spunk all over his face with the toe of my boot, he couldn't have been happier. At that moment, neither could I.

This boy is special to me, but I can't begin to describe why. I somehow feel attached in an Old Leather sense. I know he belongs to me. He considers me Old Leather, or Old Guard, although we are only seven years apart chronologically.

Old Guard refers to those that explored the world of SM Leather before the media invasion. The Old Guard passed on their knowledge and secrets by training and grooming the next generation of Leatherfolk. Nothing was written down and success to these knowledgeable men was limited. One had to prove oneself as being worthy of their time. After all, this was an investment in the exploration of the soul and not to be taken lightly. Serious business.

This boy likes the sternness of our play. He takes comfort in the rigidity and structure of knowing where he should be all the time and what the appropriate responses are that guarantee satisfaction for us both. I would allow him to experiment with the free-form style of New Leather, but he would become confused and lost in the lack of formality. Not that it does not work with some of the other boys in my immediate family, but this one likes the required etiquette of the scene. The definite preset parameters and expectations. No random options. Control.

I must admit, I function best under Old Guard attitudes and prefer that respect in my play space. Yet, in public, I am much more relaxed. Probably because most of those on the outside looking in, do not understand or they view the goings on with some confusion. Like walking into the middle of a conversation at a party and trying to figure out who came with whom.

With Old Guard, the rules are simple. All I have to do is use a code word and he assumes the proper attitude and position. Master and slave. Mentor and student. Listen and learn. Incorrect responses will be evident.

Crack!

"On your feet, boy."

He rises quickly, but stiffly. The muscles on his legs still quiver ing from the whipping and the orgasm that followed. His head is slightly bowed, never raising his eyes.

"Sir." Not a question, just a respectful response.

"Close up the dungeon and sleep at the foot of my bed, I may need to use you during the night," I said as I left the space.

As I climbed the steps from the basement. I could hear the sizzle of the candles being snuffed out and the boy was humming, satisfied. I contemplated a shower, but reluctant to remove the sweet smell of my sweat, changed my mind and headed for the bedroom. The sheets were clean and cool. I knew I would sleep well. My needs had been fulfilled, the hunger satisfied - for a while. I was vaguely aware of the presence at the foot of my bed. Sometime during the night, I awoke to find his face pressed against the sole of my foot protruding from under the blankets. I felt the stirrings of an erection, but drifted back to a contented sleep, knowing that he would still be there in the morning.

Old Leather. Images of long forgotten secrets passed down through generations. In reality, I suppose this is partly true, mankind has always applied some form of initiated passage into adulthood. Throughout history, tribes and cultures explored the same range of sensory enhancement that Leatherfolk explore today. Although Old Leather history has only been recorded since WWII, its applications have existed throughout time.

The Native American "Sun Dance" - a metaphysical leap to another plane of existence, even for just a moment - takes on a ceremony of spirituality so profound that it alters life's perceptions for the participants. Or the Crucifixion, the ultimate consensual act (after all, He knew why He was there.) And before that, the Egyptians, Romans, Mayans and a thousand other civilizations before *them*, exploring and explaining that simple primal "threshold of tolerance' and 'need'.

I also believe that my association with the men known as Old Guard has more to do with attitude than with age. Even in my mid-forties, I don't consider myself old - that is until I am around a couple of twenty-year-olds who have no concept of 'Leather', or 'community elders'. Generation gap, *big time*. But I have also met, and admire, some young men who have done their apprenticeship, and researched their needs in recognition and self-acceptance of the Old Leather attitudes and disciplines.

Unfortunately, in the great plague of the eighties, many of the most knowledgeable elders of our community have been lost. A missing generation. A break in the chain with the missing link filled in; adaptation reworked by the young men of New Leather. Men who, knowingly or not, took what they could use from the Old Guard, discarding what was of no value to their applications or interpretations, and forged a brave new view of their Leather future.

Here I stand, straddling both cultures, understanding both mind sets, yet proudly drawn to the rigid spirituality of the Old Guard.

I have come to realize over time that the love that I share within my Leather family is not restricted to a single individual. Quite the contrary. I became stunned also to discover love as non-gender specific. I mean, what could be more earth shattering than to discover an attraction that defied my parameters of sexual wants. A woman.

My God, how could this have happened? This attractive, alluring, sexually charged confrontation? Was I just imagining all this or was something deeper rising within my subconscious? Was my mother at fault for my seeking all kinds of supposed misdirection? That Freudian explanation of, "Did you really hate your mother? Was your mother too domineering?" or, "Did you have a weak father figure?"

None of the above, thank you. Love, like SM, is non-gender specific. Both are major revelations of understanding within the framework of my experiences. It can happen between two people of any persuasion, sexual-orientation, or race. Love exists. Maybe she and I had shared past lives, although, I don't believe in the traditional form of reincarnation. Of course I have no proof that it does not exist, just like I have no proof that Heaven exists (although, I think we all create our own Hell.) But I do know that we are connected on a level that neither of us understand or even wish to explain. We just accept it. Soul mates.

Our interest in, and explanation of, Leather are so similar that we sometimes scare ourselves with the need not to answer the other's questions. We also scare ourselves on a physical level, to go as far as to discuss... sex. There, I've said it. Sex with a woman. Curiosity at the least, with a compelling energy heightened by the avoidance of the discussions. After all, what would it accomplish? Our understanding of each other may be changed forever. What if it was terrible? How would we feel about each other after that? Then again, what if it was terrific? Then, what do we do? And, could I separate the act from the emotions? Now I know that whatever changes affect my life, I will always be a gay Leatherman. And I believe everything works on a continuum. I have always been the first to say, "Never say never."

Maybe I am just getting older. Not *senile*; older. But definitely mellowing. Open to more possibilities. More experiences. Isn't that how I explain to those novices that venture into my world of Leather the intricacies and depth of SM?

I understand now that I am attracted to her. Attracted to the mirror image of the use of power, of the strength and self-assurance. Quite narcissistic in a way. To recognize, gender aside, another charismatic energy. Another equal. Another Top. To be able to share and discuss, from the same perspective, without parameters, all the forces that impact our exploration of Leather/SM.

That exploration of the unknowns of SM may have been intimidating as a young man, but from where I stand now, I can still marvel at the magic it provides the apprentices of my playroom. Unfolding like a flower opening in the morning sun. And, just like the discovery of non-gender specific sexual attraction, I have come to the realization that my love expands with the relationships that are special to my 'Leather-play".

20

Of course, I love my chosen partner in ways that I am not able to define, but I also love the special boys in my life in very deep and different ways. Each for their own merits and each with their own special endearments. A power and magnetism that endlessly circles my heart like the planets circle the sun. Drawn in elliptical ways that bring our lives in line with each other during those special shared moments of SM. Cosmic man. So seventies, but accurate in a very SM way.

The ability to love more than one person at a time shouldn't come as a shock to anyone. After all, you loved your mother, father, brothers, sisters, aunts, uncles, and grandparents all at once. You never questioned your love for them, or categorized it, or measured it. It just was.

So, why do so many people have difficulty in sharing their innermost feelings with more than one person? And why should I be shocked to discover that I am attracted to a certain person sexually, gender being irrelevant. It's that Old Leather thing, I guess. That rigidity. That formality. This is the way I have defined my life. And any small warp in the bubble of understanding, from an Old Guard perspective, threatens the walls of self-confidence thrown up around me. Quite contradictory, that statement. Didn't I just finish saying that I teach my boys to explore all kinds of possibilities? I need to think about this some more.

Crack!

The timing of the invitation could not have been better. A dungeon party in Houston. A weekend of total Leather immersion. Stress relief.

The cab driver tried to look composed as he pulled up in front of the given address. A deserted street, no lights, in the industrial section. A small bulb over the door of a dilapidated warehouse. The number obviously hand drawn with fresh paint. Of course, our dress probably didn't help to soothe his nerves. Me, in full leathers, Master's Cap, Jacket, chaps, cod-piece, and boots. The boy, bare chest, shorts, boots, and collar, complete with leash and my toy bag on his lap. Wordlessly, I paid the fare and the cab was gone before we reached the door.

No lights were visible as I entered the building, followed in step by the boy. A double baffle of curtains hung inside to keep the warm glow of a thousand candles from reaching the street. I was greeted formally by the collared doorman as I produced my invitation.

*"Sir...this way please...Sir." His demeanor softened respectful-
ly as he directed me to the Dungeon Master for the evening.
The Dungeon Master was the overseer of the night's activities.
Any overstepped boundaries or disregard for preset rules would
be questioned by him. His decisions on the safety of the participants engaged in play were final and respected. Disagreements
with his decisions were taken up at a later date with the organiz-
ers. This followed the same format as parties all over the country.*

*He stood in the entrance to the play room, with his back to me,
monitoring several scenes in progress. The rules of the evening
posted on the wall beside him. They were neatly printed on an
old piece of drywall, as befitting the play space; run down, but
tidy:*

> 1. *Dungeon Master has final say.*
> 2. *No alcohol or illegal substances. Poppers okay.*
> 3. *Safe sex rules apply. Even to monogamous partners.*
> 4. *Rubber gloves, condoms ,and dams are supplied. No
>   rimming, fucking, fingering, or fisting without them.*
> 5. *Disposable containers available for needles and
>   scalpels.*
> 6. *If you want to join a scene, ask the Dungeon Master
>   to inquire.*
> 7. *Any concerns or disagreements? See Rule #1.*

*He turns at our approach and nods a greeting, a flicker of
recognition crossing his eyes. He has witnessed this dark
dance before. With a sweeping motion of his hand, he offers
me entrance to the room.*

*I step through the roughly framed entrance, mesmerized. Home.
The smell of sweaty bodies, candle wax and fear. Electric.
Spiritual. This place of reverence. Knowingly, the boy beside me
kneels and bows his head. In this place, I am complete.
Unconsciously, I place my hand on his head. Mentor, priest,
blessing this moment of personal exploration and sacrifice.*

*The room spins in slow motion as I focus on the moment at
hand. Sliding my hand down the side of the boy's face, I pull
his head against my thigh. He presses his cheek against my
leather with a moan. Such ecstasy with a simple touch. His
fears dissipate, replaced with trust as the energy passes*

*between us. Student. Acolyte. Empowered with knowledge
that something egregious is transpiring within these dilapidated
walls.*

*I bid the boy rise and, with leash in hand, approach a dimly lit
station near the center of the back wall. The floor is slightly
raised, probably a loading dock ramp, long ago boarded in.
Alter-like. Significant to the mood I am in. I survey the pattern
of hooks and bolts attached to the wall. Kneeling in front of me,
facing the wall, the boy opens the toy bag and lays out the
instruments of pleasure, lovingly smoothing the falls of the floggers and curling the whips into fine coils on the floor to his right.
We have been at this stage before and he knows my requirements; placing everything in order of usage. Tools of the trade.
Laid out with varying degrees of need or want. He removes a set
of wrist restraints, straps them on, and turns to face my boots.
Relaxed. Patient. Knowing.*

*I remove and drop my leather jacket at my feet. The boy care
fully folds it, placing it at his side. I remove my cap, careful not
to soil the brim. Sacrilege that is, to smudge the highly polished
brim. The boy avoids the brim also, and with both hands places
the cap on the jacket reverently.*

*Signaling a rotation with my wrist, the boy rises and places his
hands comfortably against the broken plaster of the wall. One
by one, I hook the snap links to his cuffs, sliding my hand down
his arms and across his shoulders in reassurance. Not a word
has been spoken, and none need be, for this is familiar territory,
well rehearsed and choreographed. Repetitive, yet new each
time.*

*Something is missing. I glance around the room. Yes. There.
A candelabra with three massive candles dripping wax down
the wrought iron like some phallic reminder of the scenes in
progress. I retrieve it and place it next to the jacket nearly folded
on the floor.*

*A light sheen of moisture reflects off the boy's back in the low
candlelight. His back is reacting with anticipation, and although
it is comfortably warm, it is not enough to produce a sweat.
I step forward, lightly stroking his back with my hand, a current
of understanding flows between us. The hunger deepens.*

There are needs to be satisfied tonight.

23

Stepping back, whip in hand, I gauge the distance to his back with a practiced eye.

Just like a scene out of Dante's *Inferno*, there is something obscenely attractive about leather. Almost like a nightmare. You wake up in a hot sweat, only to realize that you are comfortable there, that you want to remain; what happens next? Then you try to dream the dream again, but you can't go back. You can only search the edge of your experiences and try to align those events that truly reflect the satisfaction of deep needs. Dark, overshadowed needs. Magnificent unknowns that suddenly pop into your mind like snapshots. Like those sudden erections during puberty that just happen all by themselves; deep unknown needs suddenly betrayed by your subconscious, overridden by the primal urge to satisfy some unquestionable release intricately wired to your soul. And the meaningless attempts to search for logical explanations. Dark. Rebellious.

It is probably easier to explain the molecular structure of the universe. Yet, this is where my universe is at it's most logical. Tangible. Proof of my existence in the flesh. Reminders of my own mortality. And immortality.

Crack!

Delicious, that sound. Again and again.

Tears stream down his cheeks. The boy turns his head and clamps his teeth into the muscular flesh of his shoulder. Betrayed by his own need, his back gets four more. The pain becomes a friend. He grasps and relaxes in turn, floating on the first waves of endorphins. A rush. The first of many. Tonight, doors will be opened to rooms of glorious wonder, relief, and infinite wisdom. Clarity. Insight..

He uses me up. Saps my strength. Panting and bathed in sweat, I drop my arm to my side. At my feet, the instruments of our shared ritual litter the floor. My needs are feasting on these forbidden fruits. Sweet taboos. I gingerly caress his back. Hours have passed. Snapshot moments of clarity defined by the welts on this back.

Released from the wall, the boy melts into my arms. I guide him to the floor, cradling him in a tender embrace of secure assurance. I realize, for the first time, that tears float on my cheeks as well. My emotions surface and floodgates open to bathe the boy with encompassing love. Kisses with strokes of affection and accomplishment. Witnessed. Hushed whispers of approval, awe, and want are hidden behind anguished eyes of those who lack the courage to face their own needs, or are not yet ready to test their desires. The urge. Primal. Recognition of the hunger.

My universe is now in order - for a time. His needs become mine. It is time to return the gift. Aftercare.

The room returns, the candlelight softens my mood allowing me to minister all my attentions on the boy. Powerful stuff, these moments. Spiritual. Connected.

Aftercare is a lifestyle on it's own.

After all, I do not wish to damage the goods that give me so much satisfaction. Those boys whose backs feed my insatiable hunger are precious to me. Some wear their physical scar's as trophies, shown off like a variety of tattoos. Others keep them covered as personal reminders of their 'rites of passage'. But all require that emotional support and rebuilding that I call aftercare.

The exchange of power for pleasure is always consensual. Emotional scarring is out of the question, always. If I have been entrusted with the keys to the realm, I will return that trust in kind - ten fold - with the assurance that I will back up that support. Anything less is abuse.

The depth with which I play requires an equal measure of aftercare, and then some. No amount of reading the "how-to" manuals can instill that depth of responsibility. Besides, why would I not take care of my boys? I love them. And I want them to enjoy their experiences. I want them to come back. They deserve the support of their explorations. Communication is mandatory and one of the first negotiated trusts.

Hours, sometimes days, are required during that post endorphin rush. Bodily produced opiates are powerfully addictive drugs. Ask any weight lifter or long distance runner. They call it, "hitting the wall".

The personal growth and grooming of my boys is in my hands. Objects of my desire molded to my specifications. Bottoms, proud and self-assured, knowing that their needs are cared for, emotionally and physically. When I can no longer satisfy the hunger, fulfill that need, they are free. Unrestrained and capable of searching out that particular Master that can teach, rather then simply accommodate.

I have a more difficult time explaining Leather now than in those early years of exposure. I must have looked like the bantam rooster in the barnyard, strutting my colors, showing off in those brash beginnings. I could tell you anything, quotes from the writers of the time, statements of profound reasoning. I am not so sure anymore. It's deeper than the visuals now. Oh, they still have an incredible visual impact and evoke stirrings of passion and eroticism. Shock value. Erotic. Tribal. I can't even say when I noticed the change. Maybe all that bravado was just a cover. A black skinned façade.

Snapshot. There is my uncle again. Hiding behind all that masculinity and bravado. Afraid to show any kind of vulnerability. Butch with a marshmallow center. Although, I must admit that I recognized early on the armor quality of my leathers. That almost impenetrable shield that a uniform provides.

After WWII, the early gay bike clubs wore their leathers out of necessity as much as anything else. But the insignia assigned to membership carried heavy military overtones. Remnants of status and power. Whether by accident or not, still a uniform and definitely rebellious. Proudly different. But to come to the realization that the uniform did not make the Leatherman? Now that was enlightening. From 'rough 'n ready' to 'tough 'n tender'.

Maybe it was the travel, meeting others of the tribe, that brought about such insights. Getting to know men who were men, yet at the same time were capable of incredible intimacy. Whether for a night or a lifetime was irrelevant. They were whole functioning persons. A dimension that can hardly be portrayed in one-handed fiction. A community recognizing the need to celebrate it's diversity. Maybe it was the 'Plague', and the recognition that we had the power to live our lives as caring individuals. Or, regrettably, maybe it was Madonna. Suddenly, everything leather was in vogue. Everybody was copying the look. And we, or at least I, needed to reaffirm the roots of, and beliefs in, what had so profoundly changed my life.

So much for introspection. It doesn't matter what happened, the fact that it did happen is more relevant. More likely, I was balancing the leather imagery with aftercare. Parental guidance - Daddy. But, whatever the event, I wore my leathers with more purpose and responsibility than ever before. Not a crusade, but a visible signal for those searching for their own truths.

Crack!

Houston. Gray and humid. It is almost six in the morning. The cab edges down the street, searching for the number. The driver looks almost as bewildered as the previous one. I thought he was going to bolt when he spied us, but I wave several bills and he pulls to a halt. I glance back at those hand painted numbers on the door and precious memories flood past as I close the door of the taxi.

The boy looks relaxed now. He is wearing a plaid lumberjack shirt and no collar over the leather shorts. His gaze is lost on the Houston skyline visible from out hotel room. Hardly a boy, this man of thirty-something. Handsome, rugged, I like them that way. Swarthy, not pretty. And older, more secure about their sexuality. Understanding of their needs and the willingness to explore them.

As he turns from the window, I pat the bed beside me. The perfect curve of his butt excites me as he bends over to unlace his boots. A warmth spreads through my loins, watching him struggle out of the tight leather shorts. The shirt drops away and I achieve full erection viewing his welted back. Not a word is exchanged as he slips head first under the covers.

The sleep is deep and satisfying, the first in months. I shouldn't be surprised. It has been some time since the boy and I played. I haven't felt this relaxed in a long time. I roll over and sprawl out, but the boy is gone, as is his custom. He knows I need space after such an intense scene. Time to absorb the events of the evening. He also knows I like to sleep alone. Where he ended up is evident by the pillow and crumpled blanket on the sofa across the room.

He'll be back. Uncannily on time, as always.

We had given up dissecting the reason our relationship worked. We were so different from one another. He has lived with my lover and I for several years. Apart, but integral to the triad that we had affectionately come to call 3SM, a convenient play on the phrase threesome.

Although we took the SM for granted, we didn't even call it that anymore. We referred to those nights of ritual and magic as 'play' or 'Leather', totally ignoring how our uniqueness set us apart socially. We were the only long-term extended family that we were aware of locally. We had met several other multi-person relationships around the country, but our difficult and trying beginnings were modeled after no one. Finally, we settled into an accepted relationship, although not without normal disagreements.

Two Tops and a bottom. And two different Tops we were. In the early days of our relationship, the boy used to complain that we thought he was twins, as we both demanded chores or time already committed to the other. Chaos and confusion reigned until we sorted out the 'role-play' from the relationship. I remember the timid beginnings. His fear of rejection if the response he received was not what he expected. It took a while for all of us to tune into the same wave length. Except in our Leather play. There, the proceedings were formal - rigid. Old Guard. Expected. The negotiation process was almost clinical. A question period was developed after each scene purposely designed to find out what worked for each of us and what didn't.

Were the signals interpreted and understood correctly? Did an unknown or unacknowledged want surface during the scene, something that needed exploring outside the set parameters of that particular play? A need that had not been adequately addressed? But most importantly, had any emotional triggers been uncovered to create an atmosphere of suspicion or mistrust? Any past psychological scars?

Aftercare.

Crack!

I hear the key scrape the lock, and the door opens to the smell of fresh bread and coffee. He needs a shave, and his hair is tousled, but his eyes can't hide his satisfaction. Seeing that I am awake, he kneels and raises the tray. An offering. He is still in role.

"Sir." The first word he has spoken since entering the cab last night.

That one word speaks volumes. Gratification. Commitment.
I chuckle, taking the tray and swatting him playfully on the
cheek. "Now, hit the shower, we have to be out of here soon."

Mind sets. In role. Under contract. In collar.

Catchword adjectives describing men doing the work of being themselves in a Leather attitude. Why bother? Why place yourself at the mercy and control of someone else? Why defer your personal ownership, if there is such a thing?

This is the first time in history that ownership and slavery have been condemned by a civilization. Even aboriginal Americans enslaved their enemies. For all the democratic ideals throughout history, no culture has escaped enslavement in some form. Ah, but are we slaves to our own technology? For some, the high stress of balancing job, finances, and relationships are enough to send them scurrying for release. Alcohol comes to mind. I should probably mention drugs also and include how addictive money is, at least making it.

But for some special people, some who wield incredible amounts of power in their work lives, a balance is found in the role play offered in Leather as a bottom or slave. Boy toys. Age irrelevant.

Now I know that a lot of my views are met with condemnations, but I prefer to think of Leatherfolk as special people. Gifted. Able to mold their individual sensory enhancement into usable release. Definitely outside the mainstream. Or is it? Ask any sports addict why they seek such risk. Ask those construction workers who walk the 'high steel'.

The parallels are amazing. The irony of those who use Leather as an escape is that they question authority and power structures by replicating them in miniature. From a bottom's point of view, the amount of trust placed in a Top creates a safe haven within which to explore, not only sexuality, but also the fringes of all it encompasses which may be perceived as erotic.

I read that somewhere. Profound. And I never forgot it. I don't really know why it stuck. One of those turning points in my own transition from bottom to Top, I guess. All the imagination, theater, and fantasy sweeping away inhibitions within a framework of trust placed in someone else. Sensory enhancement or sensory depravation, magnifying, feeding the needs of such a release.

Coincidentally, such revelations occurred at a time when I was under-employed. Those moments of care I received as a novice Leatherman defied what I knew to be societal pressures. The stress of keeping up. Technology passing by my simple education and my low-income upbringing.

My mentor introduced me to ceremonies within our play that allowed me to grow and assertively overcome such simple beginnings. He began to educate me about myself, and from here, the rest of the world, so to speak. Enlarging the miniature and applying that to the real world. Parallels. Snapshots.

Crack!

The doorbell rang. Right on time.
I slowly edge the door open, watching the boy shuffle uneasily.

Shifting his weight from foot to foot, nervously glancing down, then at the wall, then the ceiling; anywhere to avoid contact with my shadow in the doorway. Parameters had been negotiated. Lengthy discussions led to this moment. All eroticism evaporated in the fear of rejection. What if he had overlooked something already? How forgiving would I be of the little mistakes, novice blunders? Virgin terror. Virgin excitement.

I try to ease the tension.

"Welcome. I am so pleased that you are on time."
Unsuccessful. The sound of my voice jolts him into a rigid form staring stiffly at his feet.

"Please. Step inside. The neighbors get enough amusement."

The humor escapes him. He trips over the door sill, landing on one knee, stopping his fall by throwing one arm around my knees. I almost burst out laughing, but I know he would bolt from the house, never to return, his self-esteem shattered.

I place a hand on his shoulder. He is shaking violently now. Unsure of how to proceed or what to do next.

"Calm yourself, you are doing all right. Everything we talked about is fine. Relax go downstairs to the playroom. Take your

time."

I try to make my voice sound as reassuring as possible.

"You are in good hands."

He is so intimidated by now that I can almost see his knees knocking as he races down the stairs. A little too eager to please, this boy. But if he channels all that excitement and fear and survives his own imagination, he may travel to places he never dreamed possible.

I retrieve my Coke from the coaster beside the sofa, turn on the stereo and head for the stairs. This one was going to take some time.

I silently step inside the playroom. As agreed, the boy has entered through the false panel at the back of the cell. He was facing the wall, running his hand over the bolts placed in the concrete, caressing the rough texture. Taking it all in. Tactile, feeling every precious moment build.

I clear my throat, and he instantly drops to his knees, head down, palms on the floor.

"Remove your shirt, fold it nearly, and pass it through the bars."

He had wanted to be naked, but I disagreed. This was his first time; submissive, yes, but no need to be totally defenseless. Naked. Vulnerable. In time, when the trust is complete, I will allow that surrender.

I proceed to light candles, as he sheds his shirt to the low thump of the music playing in the background. The warm glow is comforting. Turning, I pluck a hood from the wall, squat down on the heels of my boots, and toss it almost within his reach in front of the bars.

He looks stranded and his eyes plead as he sprawls and strains against the bars, willing the object of his desire to move toward him. His fingers lightly touch the edge of the leather, almost a grasp, so close, like a man dying of thirst; he can almost taste it. About to succeed, I step forward and firmly place my boot on the tip of the hood, at the edge of his fingertips. Against his will, an exasperated cry leaves his throat. So close.

He hadn't expected this. This had not been rehearsed. Sweat from the exertion ran profusely down his temples as his head drooped against the bars. The knuckles of his fist whitened as he clenched the bar separating him from the hood that was to be his salvation.

"Sir, please," he begs.

Yes. The night begins. I felt the blood pound into my groin. Sweet surrender. Reverent.

In those final moments, the boy can smell the scents that speak of a completed fantasy through the hood. Candles. Male aroma. The feel of sticky spunk on his body. Profuse thanks. Expectations surpassed.

I remove his hood in the dim light of the dungeon. Disoriented, trembling, I leave him to gather his shirt and his thoughts.

Leaning in the doorway at the top of the stairs, I flashback to other memories. Other men. Big swarthy men, with upturned collars and cowboy hats pulled down low against the buffeting mountain winds. Men on horses, dressed in leather bush chaps, heavy riding boots, spurs, and lariats. Of course, from the ground, all these images were at eye level. Marlboro men.

I had no idea that I would come to eroticize those images, those memories. This was branding time on the ranch. All the neighbors would show up on horseback, my Uncle included, for the roundup. These were exciting times, and I was glad to help. Glad to be part of all this male camraderie. I would be allowed to rope the yearlings, but I could not hold them. I was only twelve, maybe thirteen at the time. There was always some strong, dusty cowboy on hand to secure my attempts and throw the calves for branding. And I would watch as they roped each other also. Men. Games.

I found myself in the path of an old cow separated from her calf, blazing a trail to the rescue, instinctively seeking to protect it. I stood there, frozen, too frightened to move. A lariat dropped out of nowhere, violently shaking me off my feet, slamming me to the ground out of the path of a half-ton of angry beef. Choking in the dust, my arms pinned to my sides, I struggled for breath. A leather-clad hand reached out of the sky and jerked me roughly by the collar of my jacket to my feet. I squinted at the silhouette framed by the sun to recognize my uncle leaving the saddle, shaking me free of the rope. Tears tracked the caked dust on my face.

Calmly, as though nothing had happened, he turned his head and spit a wad of tobacco into the dry dirt.

"Watch yourself," was all he said. He winked and rode off.

Larger than life, he seemed right then. I thought my heart would burst as I stared after him.

I don't know why that memory surfaces just now, or if it has anything to do with the evening's events, but it has powerful imagery just the same. Important to the recent event in the dungeon.

The boy's shadow crosses the room ahead of him at the foot of the stairs. Is this how the boy had felt when I had towered over him in the dim light of the dungeon? Rescued from a collision course of conflicting emotions. Like a giant hand of fate pluck ing his soul out of harm's way.

Doubtful. How am I able to interpret his feelings about such powerful moments of release? Would words be enough? Even if he could put words to the night, would I understand his mean ings? Would I understand anything more than his basic needs?

He mounts the stairs, looks up, his face glowing, drunk with his own emotions. Relief, thanks, and understanding written all over it. He will always remember his first night of the hood.

Time now for some aftercare.

The boy kneels down in front of me, hands behind his back. As I remove the padlock from the chain collar around his neck, I drop a card on the floor in front of him.

"This list is to be learned, and repeated at the beginning of each session."

"Okay," he said, glancing in the direction of the card.

"Excuse me, boy, what did we just talk about?"

My voice carries an edge, an underlying current of condemnation.

"Sir. Yes, Sir!"

Crisply, he corrects himself, snapping back to a rigid position.

"Yes, what - boy?"

"Sir, I will be prepared, Sir."

"Yes, you will be," my voice softens. "At ease now. Make your self comfortable. You may leave when you wish."

I turn and leave him kneeling in the doorway.

He scoops up the card and begins to read the items listed.

> **Sir. The collar is to be recognized as an instrument of ownership and control, Sir.**
>
> **Sir. The collar is an instrument of submissiveness, Sir.**
>
> **Sir. The collar may be placed or removed only by the Master, Sir.**
>
> **Sir. While wearing a collar, I will not verbally respond, to acknowledge or answer others without your permission, Sir.**
>
> **Sir. The collar will always be worn with pride and honor, Sir.**

Still holding the card, he drops his hands into his lap. A look of satisfaction crosses his face, an 'I passed the test' look. He shrugs into his jacket, laces up his boots and, carefully, quietly, closes the door behind him as he leaves the house.

I stare intently into the mirror. Where has the time gone?

Cruel, time is. Betrayal by gravity. Oh, still firm, solid, this body I view, but here and there, hints of creeping age. I think I look better now than I ever did. Mature. Seasoned. Ironic. That touch of gray at the temples leading a distinguished look to my face. The military brush-cut adding authority to the gray. And those lines around my eyes, cruel or mellow, I can't tell. I'm told I have a 'game face', giving no hint to the observer of my actual thoughts. Probably due to years of self-defense, or self-preservation.

My eyes fall to the piercing through my nipples. Remnants of a sub-servient past. Gifts of pain from my teacher, mentor. I never removed them as I transitioned to Top, rather proud of them actually. I changed gauges instead, replacing the originals with heavier rings. Symbols. Personal rites of passage (I will describe those precious memories later).

My gaze drifts to my pride and joy; my arms. 'Big-guns', as body builders call them. Well earned as a teenager tossing hay-bales summer after summer on the ranch where I grew up. The left bicep encircled with a double twist of tattooe ' barbed wire. A gift to myself as a Leather com-ing-out present. Reminders of the personal fences that had imprisoned my life for so long. Also reminders of my German heritage and the out age of the 'camps', and the many gay men who perished there. But those were my reasons for the tattoo. At a casual glance, more Leatherfolk referred to the tattoo as a symbol for bondage. After all, it was on my left arm, a signal for a Top. I don't mind the interpretation; the invisible rea-sons were of no consequence to anyone but myself. Tattooed on my right bicep was a replica of a medieval hinged shackle with a ring and a bro-ken link of chain attached. Another gift to myself. Purposely thought out. Symbolism. Breaking free.

I bottom no more. My role as slave ended. My apprenticeship served. Again, another story to relate later.

I pivot in front of the mirror, to view my newest acquisition. Twelve links of chain tattooed in Leather colors with a red heart dangling from the cen-ter link all mounted across a bound man on my left shoulder. It is heal-ing well, the welts slowly dissipating.

The boy of my affections also had the bound man strategically placed on his right ass-cheek. Again, a reward. Symbolic.

From this position, I could see the tattoo on my butt; a man wielding a flogger. Memories flood into place. Memories as fresh as if they had happened yesterday. The wall I now tie young men to had once been my best friend. At times, my only support.

Crack!

It had been some time since my Master felt the need to suspend me here. By now, my thirst for the lash is unquenchable. The need to know an end was stronger than ever. I knew that this was a symbolic evening for Him. For me, the need was desper ate. I was not escaping to that euphoric plane I so deeply want- ed, to honor this occasion.

The scene was progressing. The flogger repeating it's relentless contact. The cues for assimilation lengthening, but I could not cross that threshold of deliverance that my back cried out for. The flogging stopped.

"No!" I cried silently to myself. "Not yet!"

My hunger was deep. I glanced over my shoulder, and there were tears in my Master's eyes, sorry written all over his face. This was to be an end. I could feel it. A release from my years of servitude.

"No," I prayed silently to myself, "This can't happen yet. I have not succeeded."

I do not know why, but I felt I was not there yet. With as much sarcasm as I could muster, I turned my head, stared right into his eyes, and sneered, "Faggot!"

The flogger exploded at the end of his arm. The pain was severe. The light shot through my body. Electric. Final. I went places that night I never dreamed possible. Places I needed to witness. Places one can only visit solo. Exquisite, that memory, like so many I now carry. Like the tattoo's, with their meanings not always evident or visible, but often underlying, personal. Secret. Proud.

There was no model to follow during the experimental years of our early 3SM relationship, so I will outline some of the requirements we demand- ed of our live-in boy. Now, remember, he was also part of our family rela- tionship, so a code word was set up to define periods of play as opposed to general inquiries or requests for certain chores around the property. If inquiries or questions were to be included in a contractual weekend, then they were defined or negotiated ahead of time. It sounds all very democratic, but read on. A lot of what follows came about during discussions with friends and extended family in Seattle.

> "With the agreement of both parties, Mentor and Trainee, both do agree to engage in, and abide by the following 'Rules of Conduct'. In addition, no activities will be permitted that do not fall within the range of 'Safe and Sane', applying to both sexual and non-sexual activities."

In other words, pre-negotiated parameters that protect the physical and emotional well-being of all involved. Pretty straight forward, after all, you don't want to do anything that you don't feel good about. You have the right to say "NO" without denigrating the system.

> "Mentor may cease all activities and/or halt any or all training in sessions at his discretion. Trainee may opt to withdraw from any and/or all training sessions with the understanding that any renewed or continued training is at the option of the Mentor."

So there is an 'out', for any reason, that may be exercised by either party. The catch here, for me, was the possibility of what I call a 'generation gap' or the realization that the boy/trainee may not be taking this seriously and waste my time. If the trainee (slave/boy/bottom) was withdrawing from his "formal education' for reasons that could not be discussed or re-negotiated, then why continue? Were there emotional triggers? Or, was he just uncomfortable with some aspect of the training that he was not willing to, or unable, to explain? Unquestionably, a fair amount of discussion would take place before training could resume, if at all.

> "In addition, all sessions will be conducted using agreed upon 'Safe Words/Signals'."

Self-explanatory. Although much discussion abounds as to the need for escape words or signals at all. The concept being that, at some point in a Master/slave relationship, all escape is abandoned by the slave, intimating that the Master has total ownership control. The thought is extremely Old Guard, but I believe very true.

After much discussion, basic contractual items were determined:

Novice will present himself for each committed training session ON TIME.

Novice must notify Mentor in advance of his inability to make the committed time.

Novice will present himself drug, alcohol, or enhancement free for sessions.

While in training, Novices shall not engage in any SM/BD with others. (Notice the plural use of Novice - A Top, Mentor, may have more than one trainee fulfilling his time.) Outside non-SM activities are acceptable. (In the case of a Novice, having a lover, for example.)

Novice will not engage in sexual activity prior to a training session. (Save it for the Mentor's discretion, after all, there has to be some reward. For both.)

Contractual discussions even progressed into dungeon and non-dungeon conduct. In the dungeon, a training collar was placed around the neck of the trainee by the Mentor, signifying the release of the novice's body and mind to the Mentor. This was removed by the Mentor at the end of the session.

The trainee's stance should be at parade-rest with hands behind the back, clasped hand to the wrist. The legs spread slightly apart, head down, and eyes open and averted. The trainee could speak only when asked a direct question and respond with military crispness, beginning and ending each response with 'Sir'.

In non-dungeon situations, the trainee would apprise the Mentor of any and all leather items presently in his possession and the trainee was permitted to wear only such items as allowed by his Mentor. (The thought here was that leathers, being symbols of progress, were earned.)

All agreed that the trainee was not permitted to 'flag' without permission of his Mentor. (No keys, hankies, epaulette rings or other distinctions to signify interests were to be displayed.)

In gatherings with other Leathermen, the trainee was to stand at the

Mentor's right and slightly behind. He would address everyone as Sir, unless otherwise directed, and assume a submissive stance. No verbal acknowledgment or answers were allowed without the Mentor's permission. (Here again, the discussion revolved around a 'blanket' approval to freely speak in a social setting.)

Many opinions abounded around the accidental meeting of one's Mentor socially. It was generally thought that, unless the trainee accompanied his Mentor to a gathering, he was not required to remain with his Mentor. However, permission was required to remove oneself from the presence of a Mentor. Failure to do so would certainly have consequences.

In social settings not applicable to Leatherfolk, the trainee was expected to conduct himself in a responsible manner so as not to bring dishonor or disrespect to his Mentor, himself, or all Leatherfolk.

Crack!

It was suppertime and the phone rang. It seems I can never get through a meal without interruption. That is what the answering machine is for, but I have a habit of forgetting to turn it on. It is useful for screening calls, but this time, I was glad there wasn't a mechanical voice to answer. I could hear sobbing at the other end.

"Daddy, please I need to see you, Sir, please..I must...", another emotional outburst, distress in this voice.

"Where are you?" I asked, concerned at the obvious tension in his voice.

"I..I don't know." He was quieting, the realization of his predicament was settling in.

"I'm in a phone booth."

"Give me the number, I'll call a cab. They will locate your position. Stay put. Pull yourself together, it won't be long."

The boy got out of the cab, shivering. I removed my jacket, placed it around his shoulders, and sent him into the house. He was barefoot, wearing torn, bloody jeans, and a stained T-shirt. I overpaid the driver because he wanted to record the pickup and file a report with the police.

The boy sat on the stairs inside the entrance, head buried in his arms folded across his knees, sobbing lightly. I picked him up, one arm around his shoulders, the other under his knees. He curled into my chest as I carried him up the stairs to a waiting tub of hot water.

I lightly daubed the open cuts on his butt as I dried him off. Standing outside the tub, he had his arms crossed over this chest, shivering slightly from the cool air against his wet skin.

"Now, what happened?" Purposely, I kept my voice calm and even.

"I..I just wanted to play," he stammered, choking back another sob. "He wouldn't stop! He wouldn't stop! Even when I begged... I... I...", he couldn't finish.

He was shaking uncontrollably now.

Gently I applied the antibacterial gel to the cuts. They looked like belt edges and the welts widened and rose around them. I wrapped a big towl about him, guiding him to the spare room.

"Get some rest. It's late. We'll talk in the morning."

I pulled the blanket and pillow out of the closet, throwing them on the sofa.

I waited for some time before heading off to bed. Rounding the corner, I was puzzled to see a lump in my bed. There, curled around a pillow, was the boy, sound asleep. A peaceful, relaxed look on his face.

I should have scolded him for not obeying the rules, but under the circumstances I just crawled in and wrapped my arms around him. He snuggled securely back into my chest. I would think of some way to admonish him at a later date. I may forgive, but I don't forget, ever.

I am honestly bewildered why some people put up with the shit that is thrown their way. The lack of self-esteem, self-respect, and the need to be loved or cared for, often gets in the way of common sense. Of course, late nights, cheap drinks, and depression probably account for more self-abuse than is justified. I mean, do people really need lovers or friends that constantly jeopardize their mental stability, not to mention their physical well-being, badly enough to put up with such abuse? Or is their self-hatred justified by accepting these circumstances?

Usually, those that are justifying their own inadequacies through the use of SM, find themselves out of play partners rather quickly. Most knowledgeable Tops can spot, or will avoid, these individuals, not only because they are in danger to themselves, but also because they do not want to deal with such unbalanced personalities. Ironic that I should use that term when so many non-SM people call us unbalanced. Almost an inside joke. Not really funny, though.

I guess what troubles me is that most people, even Leatherfolk, never stop to think about the difference between consensual SM and domestic violence. Leatherfolk, usually, never have to think about it; they inherently know the difference and knowingly respect each other's nature, mental and physical, even if it is unspoken.

Now don't go confusing 'SM' and 'Aftercare' with abusive confrontations followed by the honeymoon period usually associated with domestic violence. I take great care as a Leatherman to question the person I am playing with to find out about his/her reactions, mentally and physically, in establishing parameters within which to play. Safe, sane, and consensual.

An abuser rarely cares about a victim's reaction. Abuse is non-consensual manipulation, terror and power used against a defenseless victim to justify the superiority of the abuser. Abuse, however subtle, is scarring - mentally and physically. Dangerous.

Crack!

I recognized so much of myself in that hurt young man from my own childhood. Maybe that is why I reach out and talk about our Leather lifestyle so often.

One of my earliest clear memories as a child was my fear of the dark and crying myself to sleep after my father had shoved me through the attic door to cure me of my fears. I lay huddled against that door, paralyzed as all those monsters of the dark breathed on my tiny, terrified mind. Rather cathartic actually, to admit those things now. It was definitely a non-consensual, cruel

41

act.

There are many more ugly memories, but I conquered most of them with one simple stroke of manhood, although, I don't remember the details of the event leading up to it.

My father and I were standing in the barn. Something I had done or said had angered him. He was holding, or had grabbed (I don't remember), a piece of horse harness and was about to strike me with it. Reacting out of defense more than thinking about it, I reached out, grabbed his forearm, and with one hand, twisted his arm down to his side. The reality of what I had just done struck me harder than he may have and I let go of his arm.

Deliberately, I turned and walked slowly away, expecting at any moment to feel the wrath of his temper explode behind me. When I reached the door, I turned to see him standing there, arms at his side, the harness on the ground, his head bent, staring at the floor. I have no idea what he felt. Shame maybe? Weak? Possibly even afraid of me or himself? Who knows? But I do know that I removed a lot of invisible chains that day. I was sixteen and my relationship with my father changed forever.

Crack!

It took some time to pry all the details out of the boy. Probably only because there was someone there to confide in, feel safe with, did he tell his tale at all. I would like to think I was that someone, a sounding board without prejudice. But he had learned a valuable lesson and always blushes when I remind him of the experience.

I learned something too. Trust builds families and he still comes around to play now and then. But he never forgets to send a card on that date.

"So many men, so many times." A good friend, long gone now, succumbing to complications from AIDS, used to wear a T-shirt with that saying boldly splashed across his chest. I still have that T-shirt as a painful, loving memory.

Anyway, it was the saying that brought about thoughts of other men who have sought refuge in my play room. It was the play on words that struck me just now. There have not been that many men, well, a few, but certain scenes stuck out. Fragments of recollections in a sea of memories.

Ever have one of these nights where nothing can go right?

Like the night the candle accidentally fell out of the candelabra onto the bottom's chest and, although he was blindfolded, he knew what happened and started to giggle uncontrollably. All I wanted to do was to tear his chest hair out with a carpet of wax, but I ended up removing it with a small brush fire instead. Or the night I padlocked a bottom's balls to the wall without checking to see if I had the key first, and having to call a friend at three A.M. to borrow a pair of bolt cutters. Or the night I discovered a short in the extension cord of the violet wand at a most inappropriate moment. The best though, was the time the bolts came out of the ceiling with someone in the sling because I had jumped on his chest for a blow job and the support system collapsed.

It is a wonder there is anyone left to play with after all the disasters, but I have learned valuable lessons from all the experiences. I can laugh at them now, even thought they were tremendously embarrassing at the time. I learned how to be prepared, and now to be professional in carrying the scene. But most importantly, I learned how to apologize for mistakes, or errors, and still provide a good scene.

How many Leather curious people have spent years of loneliness because of the disastrous encounters, only to have their needs overcome by their fears to try again? Especially those entering our lifestyle who have had unfortunate or incompetent first time experiences? Even the best of intentions go awry. Enthusiasm can be such an unintentional culprit.

Both Leather and Leather-aware friends have blundered into public scenes and negotiations in progress, totally unaware. This happens often, especially in public, when they simply want to greet me or whomever I may be interviewing at the time. I like that word - interviewing. It sounds so formal. Depending on the setting, I will sometimes let the intrusion go, especially in public, when I have, by chance, encountered someone of interest. But if the interruption is within Leather space, I simply will not tolerate it. My Old Guard, rigid, respectful, heritage surfaces again. That is probably what gives so many Tops the reputation for being harsh, or unapproachable. So few people take in the complete picture before entering into an existing conversation. Familiarity is supposed to be comforting, but if the rejection is not intentional, then possibly just inconvenient timing.

Invasion of personal space is unforgivable, even if I'm not there. Nothing raises my ire more than someone talking to, or touching a collared bottom in role; parade rest, hands behind his back, eyes down - the signals should be clear, especially to other Leatherfolk. I have promised a couple of boys that I would make a sign they could carry saying, "No Trespassing! Private Property on Duty!" Sound selfish or insecure? You wouldn't casually walk up to a Doberman and start petting it without permission from it's Master. The same respect should be extended to a boy in my care, and hopefully, you might not get bitten. Simply put, this is my Property. If the bottom has agreed to accompany me in a collar, then he has given consent to have rules established.

Crack!

I sat in another of my favorite Leather bars called The Cuff, situated in Seattle. A number of us had congregated around the peanut barrel scooping up handfuls of nuts, tossing the shells freely on the floor, to be ground into a crunch dust on the concrete. Our boys had formed their own circle just steps away, ever mindful of their 'Tops' needs. They sat ready and willing, each anxious to out-perform the other. They were proud of their station and performed even the smallest task with great dignity and self-esteem.

I love the masculine atmosphere these bars exhibit. Amidst the smell of smoke and beer, there is that familiar aroma of Leather; some faded, some new and glistening, freshly polished, in the dim light of the high ceilings and dark painted walls.

A newcomer approached our group and introductions were made. He hugged those family members with whom he was familiar and shook the hands of those he had just met. I received a "glad to see you again" greeting with my handshake and, although I could not quite place him, I did have a feeling of recognition. He mentioned that we had met through mutual friends at Deek's, a Chicago Leather bar. He did not acknowledge or introduce the boy at this right, obviously in collar and, respectfully, a step behind his Master with his hands folded in front of him at crotch level. The boy had that enduring youthful look about him and a purposeful, knowing aura of confidence surrounded his demeanor.

The conversation resumed among the group and drinks were ordered to which the boys responded, fetching and delivering the rounds. Excusing himself, the newcomer headed for the corner near the dog-run door - so named not for the door's height, but for the style of the long patio that ran between and next to the adjacent building. I hadn't noticed the heavy chain suspended vertically from the ceiling and bolted to the concrete floor in this corner of the room until he produced a padlock and attached it to a two inch collar. He then motioned the boy toward the chain, placed the collar around his neck, and snapped the lock into place through the D-ring and one of the links. Next, he pulled a set of handcuffs from a pouch on his belt and proceeded to cuff the boy's hands behind his back outside the chain. Another pad lock appeared and was placed through a link and an attachment on the boy's belt. The boy nodded at the words whispered in his ear, but never replied. In fact, he had not said a word since enter ing the bar. The Top stepped back, surveyed his work and, sat- isfied, strode back toward our group.

He seemed amused at the obvious discomfort in which he had placed his boy. The boy briefly showed signs of anxiety which quickly dissipated, replaced with the knowledge that his Top was near. Yet no one in the vicinity paid him the slightest attention. This was nothing new to these patrons. There were hooks, rings, and chains all over the building for such public displays. The only outlet for many who desired such fantasies. For the novices of the community, this provided an exciting, erotic glimpse at the reality and formality of a culture.

The Top maneuvered himself into a position that would allow a view of his property and resumed his conversations. By now, my curiosity was aroused as to the intent or culmination of the wit- nessed events. Was this a public humiliation scene? Possibly a 'rite of passage'? Was it part of a larger fantasy, with the public display acting as sexual foreplay that so often manifests itself in verbal terms prior to play? Or, was this just fun, of and for it's own sake, consented to beforehand? My mind was playing all kinds of games with these visual puzzles. Could this be punishment for some act of wrongdoing, real or perceived, on the part of the bot- tom? I smiled at the exquisite thought.

The Top noticed that I had ignored the conversation around me, absorbed in thoughts of the boy on the chain. Leaning over my shoulder, he said, "I'll let him stew awhile. I told him he'd be made available to whoever I found interesting."

"How perfect!" I thought, "What this boy must now be experi-

45

encing! Was he excited by the notion that his Top was picking out someone for him to serve, or service, be it another Top or a bottom? Was he terrified at the thought that his Top might actually go through with it? Pushing boundaries. Questioning consent. Tapping unknown fears."

The Top could work the room knowing that his boy was right where he had left him - on display - and that, with every glance or nod in his direction, his Top could watch the panic rise and subside in the bottom's eyes. Every word would leave questions in his mind, "Is this the one? Or is there more than one? Or worse, none of them." Fear is a wonderful tool.

An obviously intoxicated Leatherman stumbled through the door of the dog-run, and supported himself against the wall near the chained boy. I felt the Top stiffen beside me, on alert. I was also conscious of the boy's reaction to his helpless predicament. The Top was in motion, shifting through our circle, aware of the impending catastrophe. The drunk leered and reached forward, grabbing a handful of nipple and flesh and twisting violently. As the Top reached full stride, a hand shot out, choking off the laugh emanating cruelly through the alcoholic haze. The drunk's eyes bulged in shock as the hand lifted him off his feet, slamming him against the door frame he had only moments ago entered. His beer shattered on the floor and he clawed at the fist on his throat choking off precious air as the momentum carried them both through the doorway to the narrow patio. Few even noticed the altercation, it had happened so fast. A slight scuffle ensued out side and the Top emerged in the doorway, straightened his jacket, and patted his boy on the butt reassuringly. The boy smiled weakly and nodded his thanks, relief, and love shining in his eyes.

Calmly, as if he had just gone to relieve himself, the Top rejoined the conversation, again positioning himself where he could keep a watchful eye on his property. Knowing whispers and nods of appreciation and respect slowly circulated the room. I could feel the power emanating from this man and the respect being paid by those around us. He was so very protective and exuded confidence and self-assurance - all qualities that I admire and emulate.

I have been referring to my play-room a lot, so maybe I should explain my approach to it's value as personal space. It is my sanctuary. A place for ritual and ceremony. Any entrance to this space is by invitation only, and usually, this is forwarded to those with the same general interests in the activities I explore. The space is not large, so a wide variety of interests cannot be accommodated.

If more than one person is invited, I consider it polite, but not necessary for them to call and inquire if there is a need to contribute to the party in the form of special equipment, for example, food or maybe even such basics as candles. I consider it not only rude, but quite inappropriate to show up at a play party dressed in dungeon wear. Street leathers are quite acceptable, but I have to live in the neighborhood and a cod-piece and hood just fuel the neighbor's anxiety.

Although soundproofing is not a problem in my space, I recommend that bottoms supply their own gag. There is no need to disrupt other scenes in progress. I insist that any implements that are borrowed be cleaned and set back on their shelves. And I expect, out of consideration, that if they have not been to my space before, they ask about the guidelines and what are allowable sports. Times and moods change and some parties are more conducive to certain activities than others. For example, water sports or blood sports may not fit the theme of the evening or may be uncomfortable for some players.

The rules of my space are pretty straight forward:

- Play safely and within your limits regardless of the environment. Peer pressure and available equipment does not justify experimenting or overstepping your known abilities.

- Do not touch what is not yours without the permission of the owner. This applies to Tops or bottoms.

- If this is your first invitation, ask about a change room, bathrooms, and emergency facilities.

- Make your scene intentions known and ask if there may be objections to a particular scene.

- No drugs or alcohol!

- Do not gawk or linger too long when observing an activity. This may be considered voyeurism and, unless the scene was set up for public viewing, it may destroy the mood.

- Don't ever interrupt a scene. If you have a question, mentally note it, and seek out the participants later. Most will impart information and explain the details about why they are involved in such an activity.

- If you wish your slave/bottom/boy to experience something out of your range of expertise, approach a Top with the desired skills and ask if He could spare the time allowing your bottom to experience his particular craft. Even if the answer is "No", your request will be treated with respect.

- If you are a bottom wearing a locked collar approaching a Top, be sure to explain your request using, "…with the permission of my Sir or Master," or the Top may not acknowledge your presence. After all, you are someone else's property. A Top, after listening to your request, may wish to speak to the Master/Top/Mistress directly. This does not belittle or demean the bottom, but helps clarify the meaning or choice of words used in the request and also shows respect and acknowledgment of his Owner. Most problems can be eliminated simply by observing more experienced Tops and unintentional interference can be avioded.

I purposely choose to explain all of this with the use of multiple scenes in the same space. But the rules apply as well to private, one-on-one fantasies.

Crack!

I took a deep breath and my heart pounded adrenaline through my veins. Every muscle in my body was frozen, every nerve alert as the clamp was placed over my nipple.

"This will restrict the blood flow and help deaden the nerves," he said calmly, "and it probably hurts worse than the actual piercing."

I drew another breath, not at all reassured.

The hollow needle approached my nipple. I was totally mesmerized and found that I could not look away, even if I wanted to. It felt strange, watching a foreign object invade my body, like watching those slow motion movies with bullets or arrows splashing through pieces of fruit or soft wood. Suddenly a soft, white hot, electrical shock wave of delayed awareness ripped through my body. As the needle exited the other side like a knife through butter, a crimson pearl formed around it's edge. The clamp was removed. The nipple stiffened and stood erect as blood pumped into the flesh around it, solidly gripping the intrusive rod. Strange, there was no pain - yet.

"Relax." He said, "I just have to slip in the ring."

The arches of my feet tingled as they relaxed. I had been so unaware of the tension in my body. Everything from my butt cheeks to my shoulders cried for relief. I knew I would have marks on my wrists after this scene. I was strapped face out to the flogging wall I knew so well.

My Master stood just out of the circle of light thrown by the candles. His arms were folded across his chest in satisfaction and excitement glittered in his eyes. He stepped forward into the light and slowly withdrew the needle, a steel ring in it's hollow end to replace it. The needle was gripped so firmly by the flesh it had penetrated that I was reminded of those early gladiator movies, where the victor would place his foot on the slain captive to remove his sword. Such seminaries were attributed to my now captive nipple. A trickle of blood flowed freely and, with a gloved hand, my Master traced red patterns across my chest. I started to float as the first sweet, exquisite wave of pleasure rushed in, replacing that the searing throb.

He stretched the rubber gloves from his hands, obtained fresh ones, and snapped them into place. As he approached the other nipple, my toes curled in spite of themselves and the clamp tightened over my defenseless flesh. Another ecstatic, light-headed rush crept up the base of my skull. Again I felt the needle's bite, only not quite as severe when the clamp was removed. Possibly due to the activated endorphins already in my system.

I looked down. Two exotic, sparkling circles protruded from my chest. They looked tribal. Resting my cheek against the coolness of the wall, I started to laugh and then cry, both at once. Time lost all relevance and I remained afloat in a sear of emotions as I surveyed my new gifts.

I flipped to Page 94 of the *Leatherman's Handbook* (Larry Townsend). It was thumb-worn and ragged from so many one handed readings. Never before had I come across such a fantasy. In fact, the action on those pages had never occurred to me, but once introduced, I couldn't release those images. And, so accidentally I had come across it, that its impact was probably all the more powerful. Erotic? Hell, yes! Both decadent and degrading, but inexplicably hot. Few other acts had spurred such visceral reactions in me, such a silent stirring in my soul.

Communion. That is the word I have been searching for. Rewarding. Satisfying. Nearly as close for me to the rapturous high attainable from the delivery end of my whip or that frozen-in-time eternity of agonizing pleasure just prior to orgasm. Maybe it was just the idea that such an act was playing on the edge of forbidden civilized behavior. Stepping across the line, so to speak, to claim or justify that rebel image that had haunted my memories since childhood. The ultimate act of dominance or submission, depending upon the interpretation of the need. The ultimate taboo. Piss. Water sports. That sweet forbidden release. Baptism. Now there's a contradiction, though somehow, fitting.

Crack!

It was Saturday night and the bar was crowded. The shaggy Horse was named after the shag carpets that used to line the walls. The carpets are long since gone, thankfully replaced with the original brick walls. No one ever leaned against those walls for fear of what might be living in them. Not to mention the foul, lingering stench of smoke and beer.

I leaned against the railing of the second floor, overlooking the dance floor below. Above me, the air conditioner circulated a semi-fresh breeze through the dense smoke-filled room.

Saturday night. Leather night.

The bar was filled way over capacity and sweat stained bodies juggled for position, maneuvering in and out of the lineups for the washroom or drinks at the bar. A young man had caught my eye earlier in the evening. I was almost annoyed at his obvious attempts to stay in my line of sight. He was determined, this one, but I was here to socialize with friends, not cruise. But he wouldn't give up and it became a game to see how long it would take him to make a move. Would he overcome his fear of rejection and how appropriately would the introduction proceed?

I eventually lost sight of him and though he had given up. But my interest was now roused and I glanced around the room and saw him standing at the bar ordering another drink. Then I forgot about him for a while and stood and chatted with my friends. Turning, I stepped away from the circle to head for the washroom and abruptly bumped into someone. About to apologize I realized that this was the same young man and he had been standing behind my right shoulder, probably for some time, holding two beers at chest level.

He offered me one. "Sir, for you," he said, a rush of insecurity flooding his eyes.

My response was more automatic than thought out, "I'm sorry, I don't drink."

Rejection flooded his face. I caught the look and myself, and immediately responded, "But you can get me a Coke while I take a piss," and pushed my way through he crowd.

He was nowhere in sight when I returned and I thought he had been frightened off or lost interest, but no sooner had I resumed my position at the rail, when a hand thrust a glass of Coke toward me. He positioned himself as close to my right as possible, almost beaming with pride that he had accomplished his task so quickly in such a crowded place. I glanced in his direction and nodded my thanks then ignored him as I rejoined the conversation of the circle.

Sometime later I became aware of his presence, fidgeting nervously, shifting his weight fromfoot to foot. The beers had finally taken their toll on his system. He badly needed to relieve himself. If he had disappeared to use the facilities, I probably would never have taken any notice, but the fact that he stood there waiting for acknowledgment of this predicament intrigued me. Was he purposely waiting for my reaction? Well, he was going to get one now that he had piqued my interest.

"Sir, may I use the washroom?" he requested.

"No," I said flatly.

I thought to myself, I wonder how interested this one is and how obedient he can be.

"Can you take orders?" I asked.
"Yes, Sir, if you say so, Sir."

"Good, I said, "Piss your pants."

His eyes got big, he swallowed hard, opening his mouth as if to protest, and consciously closed it again.

"Yes, Sir," was all he said, his face reddening with embarrassment.

I glanced down to watch him ball his fists at his side, fighting back his discomfort.

A small wet patch appeared in his crotch, spreading down the inside of his jeans to his chaps. Slowly a small pool formed on the floor at his feet.

I got an instant erection and the whole intent of the evening changed at that moment. I reached for my wallet, retrieved the check stub and extended it toward the young man.

"Get my jacket, boy," I ordered.

My voice was husky, heavy with excitement.

"Yes, Sir."

A grin spread across his face as he headed for the coat check at the front of the bar.

Knowing at once that the world is somehow different, that perceptions are altered toward all that applies to our unique, Leather understanding. Now I know that watersports have absolutely no appeal to some. Also, it may have no relationship to SM for other enthusiasts. But for me, it was another turning point. An act that, devoid of any environment related to SM, could be as magical or powerful as any dungeon scene I had encountered.

Maybe my timing of the discovery was just right. Maybe I would not have interpreted this meaning of the gift had I come upon it at any other time in my life. After all, I was discovering a world of possibilities that had never before occurred to me. Whatever the reason, the discovery was profound and definitely adds to my repertoire of enjoyable experiences to be shared.

Voyeurism is to watch and learn. It is exciting to watch a skilled Master put a willing bottom through his paces. Even if I have no interest in exploring that particular craft, the ability to draw parallel meaning from such an exercise is revelation. I have discovered other interests that I had never before considered under such circumstances. Voyeurism is one-handed satisfaction at the least, and erotic education at it's best.

There isn't much the three of us haven't tried, whether individually or as a team of two Dad's and a boy. Although some things don't interest me, there is a growing sense of voyeurism. But then, my whole life has been one of watch-and-learn. As a carpenter, my skills were well honed under the tutelage of an old European craftsman. He taught me pride in my work and, no matter how simple the piece, I left my signature on it. Not with my name always, but certainly with my accomplished style.

Creativity through my hands. I can trace my family of craft and trades men back to the early 1600's in Hamburg, Germany. Ironically, the first records of the family tree were kept by a cobbler, a leather craftsman. How coincidental that I should find such solace in the feel and texture of the hides I mold into personal pieces of expression. So, it seems that I have translated all my inherited gifts into one convenient package. All those generations of creativity narrowed to a fine point. Like standing between two railway tracks and watching them merge into one in the distance.

There is strength in the knowledge that each rail or facet of creativity is part of a whole, and yet somehow, strong enough to stand alone. Reminders of backup electrical circuits that fail. A replaceable supply of alternatives. Creative outlets, each selected and triggered by a different set of response. My view of the Dungeon Master parallels these thoughts. He becomes director, psychologist, props manager, and scriptwriter, all in one. This fully rounded individual enables the bottom to explore a full range of experiences, emotions, and fears with total support and confidence. Mentor and student. And maybe that is why I feel that my education as a Top is never complete. There is always some applicable piece of information cropping up to spark new approaches and explanations.

Crack!

There we were, my lover and I, standing inside the dungeon door knowing the two boys were naked, on their knees, awaiting our call. Two Masters, allowing tension and excitement to build on the other side of the door. Candles had been lit along the whipping wall and the bondage board had been suspended in the middle of the room. My lover wore a raunchy old jock-strap while I was naked except for a hood and boots. He held a blindfold in one hand and a bottom's hood lay on the floor at my feet.

I stood in front of the whipping wall, arms across my chest. He glanced in my direction, I nodded and he opened the door.

"Boys," was all he said.

The intonation in his voice was clear. The boys, not daring to look up, crawled into the dungeon on their hands and knees. No particular order was chosen; it was not needed. The first boy through the door crawled the full length of the room to kneel at my feet. The second boy stopped just inside the doors, not quite sure where to position himself. His Master closed the doors and snapped a padlock in place as an involuntary shiver ran through the boys' shoulders at the sound. That sound had a ring of finality to it.

I grew hard as I watched him place the blindfold on his boy. Mistaking my erection for a signal, my boy started to nuzzle my crotch. Wrong. I pushed his head down to my boots and, with out a word, he started to lick. It felt good, almost massaging my feet through he leather with his tongue. I leaned back against the wall and feasted on these sights before me, the warm glow of the candles throwing macabre shadows against the wall. Voyeurism. So very erotic.

"Rise. Turn, step back, sit," He said, guiding his boy to the bondage board.

Slowly, he manipulated the boy onto his back and started to do up the restraints. One at the waist first, then three on each arm and two on each of the boy's legs. Special horseshoe-styled restraints were placed over the boys feet and secured to the chains supporting the weight of the bondage table. Circling the table, he pulled a small leather pillow off its place on the wall and slid it under the boy's head.

"Don't make yourself too comfortable," He said, "but then it wouldn't last long anyway." A deep chuckle followed.

The boy tensed involuntarily. A violet wand was retrieved from it's resting place and plugged into a convenient outlet above the imprisoned boy. As the first charge of static electricity was applied to the inside of the boy's thigh, he jerked to the limits of his confinement. An involuntary moan, more than from surprise than pain, escaped his lips.

"What did you say, boy?"

"Sir, thank you, Sir," replied the boy through clenched teeth.

I was so lost in the scene unfolding before me that I had forgot ten about the boy at my feet who by now, having not been told otherwise, was licking his way up the inside of my thigh, seeking the object of his desire waving in the air above him. I did not acknowledge his whimper of disappointment as I pushed his head back to my boots.

The electric wand was replaced with, of all things, a pattern cutter. A small wheel styled spur placed at the end of a curved handle. The response he was extracting from the boy was amazing. The boy's body jerked and spasmed at the slightest touch of this small tool, his fists clenching and releasing as the tool was applied or withdrawn at random intervals.

Pulling him up with a dripping wet boot under his chin, I raised the boy's head to my crotch. He eagerly went to work, almost starving and insatiable. I relaxed into the immense pleasure, rolling my head back against the wall, eyes closed, lost in my own thoughts of the scene surrounding me.

When I looked again, the spur had been replaced with tit-clamps and clothes pins. The clothes pins were lining the insides of the boy's thighs and ball-sac. This was more than I could bear to watch. The bottom's hood on the floor at my feet was of no use now. Need had replaced the visuals.

Roughly, I pushed the boy away as I reached for a condom. The boy, now on the floor at my feet, didn't have a chance to protest, not that he would have anyway.

55

"Mean, tough, cream-puff."

A trans-gendered friend called me that at a workshop one time. I didn't know whether to laugh or spit nails. But in the context of the larger conversation, I knew what he meant by it. We had been discussing a whipping demonstration that we both taken part in. One of the comments I had made referred to a bottom being willing to skin their knees within the context of certain scenes. I had used that phrase in reference to the miscalculations that occur during play. A sort of no-fault policy due to the fact that accidents are more likely to occur in spaces that have little light, low ceilings, too loud music, or too crowded. Also, distractions of any kind can momentarily warp a person's sense of timing or distance. All of this related specifically to a special perspective with the use of whips. My point was, if I throw a thousand strokes with a single-tail whip, I am bound to miscalculate one or two. Shit happens.

The "mean, tough, cream-puff" comment was made in relation to my ensuring that my bottom was okay, both emotionally and physically, after my mistake. The fact that I actually cared about my bottom's well-being and acknowledged it drew various negative responses from the audience. To some, I became 'too-real', meaning that my ability to 'feel' got in the way of their fantasy. Some wanted truly sadistic scenes in which the bottom viewed the Top as an uncaring power figure. A valid point too. These fantasies are needed by some and, I admit, there are times when I enjoy them also. But to the majority of the audience, I became 'more real'. My ability to acknowledge an error gave them another dimension to the term Top. I could provide a safe and trustworthy place to explore their fantasies, within the confines of their submission. A place to let go knowing they might trip but I would catch their fall.

A "mean, tough, cream-puff" is a rough exterior with a marshmallow center and a great analogy of most Leatherfolk in my opinion. I have never met more passionate and caring people in my life.

As a Top some of the most rewarding scenes I have participated in the have evolved from emotional bonding rather than the physical play inherent to domination/submission roles. I value a bottom who is creative, spontaneous, and objective. I do not wish a doormat. After all, someone who can think for themselves also pushes my creativity and limits. It is the respect shown me as a Top that carries weight and has the most value emotionally, in or out of the playroom. The emotional status of my bottom is of utmost importance. If we are playing in an unhealthy environment, then we are inviting disaster. Negotiation and responsibility are appropriate to individual sessions.

One thing I have not mentioned yet is down time. If a contract has been negotiated for an extended period of time, I do not feel that I have to monitor a bottom's behavior one-hundred percent of the time. Not only do I value a self-thinker, but both the Top and bottom need some down time to recharge the creative batteries that refresh the play. Not time out, but just a toned down period that allows readjustment or re-evaluation of the contractual needs. Specifics can sometimes become side tracked or warped out of perspective if the period of intensity is too long. Not that some players do not wish this depth of play. For example, a weekend of intense bondage and the ability to play for a lengthy period, for me, requires tremendous focus. It is exhausting, especially if the sexual energy has been spent early on. A change of pace helps rebuild interest. I receive tremendous pleasure in being able to increase or relax the intensity of an extended period of play, contractual or not. Mind games help keep the bottom on his toes.

The ability of a bottom to spontaneously react to similar scenarios in a variety of ways, within the parameters of respect and acknowledgment, allows me to be more creative in discovering what works for both of us during a scene. If I receive the same monotone response to a variety of manipulations from a bottom, then either he is not relaxing into a scene and allowing his reactions to talk for him, or I have failed to extract the correct information about what the expectations of the scene were for both of us.

Even through clenched teeth, a difference can be intimated just by volume. The exception to this being if the bottom displays a "this-is-a-test" attitude to discover what it takes to make a Top abandon the scene. The 'you-couldn't-get-a-response-so-I-win' attitude that some bottoms exhibit. Well, they usually get a response from the Top they were not expecting. Translate that anyway you wish. I have two words for pushy bottoms - duct tape. I have to insert here that some of the boys I have played with repetitively use this tactic to see what my limits are. Well, boys, it's not nice to test Daddy's patience. And to be fair, if I am not getting the responses I expect, maybe our needs just aren't meshing. Mood swings and expectations are influenced by many factors both before and during a scene. The trick is to know when it is not working and call it off rather than perform a mercy-fuck just to save face.

There are times when the bottom just puts out and shuts-up, especially if Daddy is in the mood to mete out some long-remembered act of retribution. "Forgive but never forget" is my motto, and it comes in very handy.

Crack!

The ultimate sin and I caught him in the act.

I work early, as does my lover, and we trust that the daily chores around the property will be taken care of at some point through out the day. Now, we have never set particular limitations, except for the 'no masturbation' rule, upon our boy. There are certain expectations and they are usually accomplished within the required time frame.

One morning, I ran an errand for work and I swung past the house to kill a little extra time. Assuming the house was empty, I bounded up the stairs to my bedroom only to find, in the middle of my bed, curled up in the warm spot I had only recently left, wrapped around my pillow, was our boy.

He didn't move or breath, then slowly, one eye opened.

"Hi?" , he said, with a quiet voice, several octaves higher than normal.

I had never seen such guilt expressed so vividly.

I looked right past him, as though I had never seen or heard him. I saw a long sleeved shirt slung across the trunk at the foot of my bed.

"There it is," I muttered, barely audible, using the shirt for an excuse, totally forgetting the reason for my return. I retrieved the shirt and disappeared down the stairs, out the door and off to work again. I was laughing so hard that I had tears rolling down my cheeks and I wondered what he was doing now.

Was his heart pounding in fear at the though of getting caught? Was he scrambling into clothes for fear I may return and demand an explanation? Was he laying there, clutching my pillow in hor-ror of the consequences, maybe hoping I had not seen him? After all, I had not even acknowledged his presence.

Still laughing, I though, "File this one for future use - at the appro-priate time, of course. Ah, sweet fate. I'll let him squirm for a while. He'll relax eventually. I"ll bet he tip toes around his duties and the conversation for a few days though. Besides, time is on my side and I never forget."

The only risks worth taking are the ones with the largest unknowns. Obviously, if the conclusions were known, there would be no risk. I don't believe in little risks either. To me, this means that the chance of failure is so minimal that the loss is tolerable - unless we are talking about money, of course. I am not talking about gambling either, at least not in a monetary sense. I would like to think that I deal in risk as a learning experience. The chance to further my knowledge about me. Now, don't take this as a signal for edge play or sexual roulette, but as an option to create a parallel to life.

Leather is not just about SM; it is an avenue within which to explore the entire world. I am not trying to be cosmic or psychological in a Freudian way, just stating that I do not want to be one of those folks that regret their missed moments, lamenting, "I wish I had done that when I had the opportunity," or, "maybe I should have taken the chance."

I believe, in the large scheme of things, the bigger unknowns usually have the greatest rewards. Chalk it up to experience. Hopefully this is not misconstrued as being impetuous but, when was the last time you were driving somewhere and, out of the blue, you turned left instead of your usual route just to see what was on the way, only to discover that this was a more interesting or varied road? In the long run, what have you got to lose? I think the saying goes, "Experience is what you get when you didn't get what you wanted." Hell, some days just getting out of bed in the morning is a risk.

All too often, the limitations placed on play are the same barriers we subconsciously place on ourselves in everyday life. No one likes to think of themselves as self-limiting. At the same time, I have overheard a lot of people say, "Oh, I can't do that". Why not? I mean, maybe not instantly, but work up to it. Like easing into a cup of hot coffee, too hot at first, but slowly it becomes bearable, then comfortable, and pretty soon, you have to add more hot water. Just like SM.

I have also learned of a dark side to the risks. I could never have anticipated it. It scared the hell out of me actually. A bottom I had tied to my whipping wall was totally freaking out and lost in the absolute terror of his imagination. What had sent him into such a panic I did not know at the time. Although, looking back, I can probably guess what triggered it and sent him beyond what he was prepared for emotionally.

I may not have given him enough support throughout the beginning stages of the scene. But, in my own defense, I had proceeded the way he had negotiated. In retrospect, I should never have begun the scene but all this was new, raw, and exciting to both of us. He was young, brash and the scene was set by his limitations. I was to supply the required amount of fear to make it work. So, I jumped right in, too deep and too fast. I never asked him why this was important to him and no discussion ensued regarding what needs might be satisfied for us both.

I know better now. I know what to ask, how to ask it, and how to deduce the subtle answer about what was not said as opposed to what actually was. It was a hard way to learn the lessons but I suppose it's inevitable. Mistakes generally occur because of eagerness to be part of a scene. In this case, I had been thinking with my dick instead of my head. Experience is the best lesson.

I can't begin to describe how all of this fits into my world. It is extremely hard to compare what happens in my Leather space to my work place. The language we all use to communicate is borrowed, adapted, and labeled with special meaning to become applicable to the Leather culture. Words are still words, but some have dual meanings and carry more power under circumstances for which the original meanings were not designed. Power transference and attitude aside, I have learned to exist in the larger social world with much more confidence because of my Leather lifestyle. I am more comfortable with who I am as a person. My world fits me now. I have not compromised or sacrificed anything to fit it. But I have adapted to the pressures more easily because of my Leather.

Almost everything we do in our everyday lives involves that ability to negotiate. Even an act as simple as going for lunch with a co-worker depends on the ability to interact socially. Where to eat? Fast food or sit down? What to wear? All involve the unconscious ability to negotiate. And, just like life, Leather is a microcosm of the real world. Of course, to some of us, Leather *is* the real world and work just gets in the way.

It boggles my mind to think that so many people have difficulty communicating their needs or wants when the topic of discussion just may include an erotic connotation. After all, these same people have no trouble telling the waiter to hold the onions, or substitute the gravy for salad. My Leather taught me one very important fact: communication is not just talking, it is also observing.

Good communications skills - more to the point, good *listening* skills - allow me to disseminate information and express ideas that ultimately lead to my objective, whether that objective is buying a car or negotiating my way into someone's pants. I remember scolding a bottom and telling him that there was a reason he had two ears and one mouth. His wrong reply was, so that I had something to hold onto while he gave me a blowjob. He was difficult, but he got over it - with a little help from the welts on his back.

I am passionate about communicating clear intentions and expectations; almost clinical. No misrepresentations here, but I always listen for those comments and answers that allow a willingness to explore or expand upon the limits imposed. My ability to listen had been many years in the making. And often, I learn more from what has not been said than what has; body language is an important communicator.

At work or play, people assess your meanings through a combination of sources. Hand movements speak of intent, but the eyes, the eyes show both trust and insecurities. We all learn these things as children. I can remember being scolded many times by my mother's eyes. Words were not necessary and retribution always followed. I do not mean social-sub-servience is a must - we all have an opinion and I am quite forthright about some of mine. Also, what works for me many not be applicable for anyone else, but if I am speaking, then I am not listening. Too many people like to hear themselves talk because it makes them feel important. Listening allows me to change my mind about a willingness, or unwillingness, to advance the conversation with someone to whom I am attracted. It is difficult to retract an invitation to play without casting some suspicion as to why I may have changed my mind.

I recall negotiating for an extended period of time with a bottom. I asked him to select a couple of items from the toy wall. I then suspended him in bondage, gathered up all the toys he had chosen and put them in a box. "Now then," I said, "these are not the toys we will be playing with." I received a look of absolute panic and excitement.

I had been able to discern from all the conversations that the items he had chosen were within his comfort zone. I had also determined, correctly, that this was not what he was after; what he had subconsciously asked for was an expansion of his limits, to conquer certain fears and to explore. At the same time, had I not been absolutely sure about his interest, the evening could have been disastrous. Many scenes have gone awry because of misinterpretation. For this reason, the ability to listen, as well as the ability to ask the right questions without tipping your hand are crucial to success.

I would hope that this approach does not apply to everyone. We are individuals with out own reasoning abilities and interpret available information differently but the results are usually the same. I must admit however, that I listen more closely now to what is being conveyed. Not that I have become picky about my play partners, just a little more selective about the needs we will be sharing during a scene.

Crack!

I was at the AA Meatmarket in Chicago for the International Mr. Leather weekend. There really is no way to fully explain this yearly trek to Chicago except to say that five thousand or so men in one city for a Leather weekend is quite spectacular and empowering. Not to mention its impact on tourists and hotel staff.

As a special request, I had made arrangements to meet one of my boys from San Francisco for a social weekend. He had met someone he wished to Top. A fellow from Seattle, whom we had both met on a previous holiday, had wished to bottom for him. I was delighted. In my view, this is what my role as mentor is all about - I was passing along to the next generation all that I had been able to convey. And now, I had been asked to witness this ascension, this graduation from bottom to Top.

The AA was packed and so condensed that from a ceiling view, we must have all looked like salmon squirming around on a spawning run. I worked my way into the back room. One small bulb of a low wattage hung over the circular bar. More light was splintered over the crowd from the television hung in the corner than from that bulb. I picked a spot against the brick wall, out of the traffic circle. That endless tour of shirtless, sweaty men that circulate the bar on the move constantly. The AA Meatmarket - aptly named, I thought.

The sexual tension in the room was so thick you can cut it with a knife. The want and hunger shone in the eyes of so many men. Rancid and sweet need exuded out of every pore and mingled with the sweat. There was a sense of urgency in the air, mixed with the dense smoke wafting down from the two fans hanging from both ends of the room. Eventually, my eyes adjusted to the low light and I was able to watch for my friend.

I chuckle as I think about him with a sense of fatherly pride. The boy had grown. I need a drink but I am not willing to lose my spot to the swirling circus of flesh. I'll wait. Several familiar faces float past, nodding in recognition. This is my fifth year at this event, almost an old home weekend. And this is one of the great social weekends of the year for Leatherfolk. A reunion. One that encompasses all that is good and bad about our community.

I have often heard the statement; "You guys just stand around and look miserable, you don't have any fun when you go out."

What's the definition of fun? Getting drunk until you puke or dancing until you drop? Or drugs? Now, there is one that just does not make sense to me; putting a chemical in your body to make your mind think it likes you so you can have a good time all by yourself. Substance induced self-esteem. And some people call SM silly and make-believe. But for someone who is clean and non-drinking, I guess my attitude is to be expected. Besides, I have more fun watching these people make absolute fools out of themselves, telling and laughing at jokes and each other as they get sloppy and think that they are being hilarious. Well, they are, but the really funny part is - they're the joke. And I don't have a hangover in the morning. I can stand against the wall all night, totally entertained, and not have said a word. Drugs and alcohol are not the only crutch. I also watch people use SM as a substitute for self-esteem, performing any act necessary to get a little attention. Even if it is negative attention, it's better than no attention at all.

The looks on those faces swirling around the bar are enough to entertain me all night. The music seems to increase in volume, rhythms guiding the gyrating masses, the din of conversation lowering under the weight of the music, communication becoming eye contact only. The hunt has started. Needy eyes, glazed eyes, come-fuck-me eyes, eyes that were begging just for that masculine touch against their skin at any cost. The want was so evident that it scares off most with its pleading and eagerness. Few eyes make contact with mine. It is the honesty in my eyes, I think, that is intimidating to most. Nothing superficial about the questions in my eyes, "What are you really looking for?" and, "Are you prepared to be honest in return?" No hidden agendas here. It is that game face again that I have been accused of wearing so often. Naked trust questioned at a glance. "Are you willing? Will you bare your throat to the wolf with the red roses?" They glance away.

I still need a drink. I'll have to trade off my parking spot to quench my thirst or at least until another spot becomes vacant. Maybe I should snag a boy with an open collar? No. He might mistake that for a signal of interest. My gaze is attracted to a wave in the crowd and I recognize an old acquaintance from Florida. A Master that I had met several years ago in San Francisco and had bumped into several times at events like this. I watched him thread his way through the crowd until he was within reach and clamped a friendly hand on my shoulder. He wedged his way in front of me, smiled, and stuck out his hand in greeting.

"Long time," he said, solidly shaking my hand.

"Yeah," I laughed, "last year, same time, same place."

For the first time, I noticed a fit young man standing behind him wearing a collar. The leash end was in his mouth and he clasped a dog dish tightly in his hands.

"Another new one?" I questioned

"They don't seem to last long," he winked and smiled.

"I need a drink and probably a piss too if the line isn't too long. Hold my spot? You want another beer?"

He nodded a decline over the offer for a beer never even looking in the slave's direction, just subtly pointed a finger to the ground at his side. The boy was very astute. I hardly noticed the gesture. The slave dropped to his knees against the wall I had just vacated.

"Thanks, I could be awhile."

"No rush," He replied as I stepped into the flow of traffic.

As I disappeared into the crowd, I saw him pour a little of his beer into the dog dish from waist level. Some splashed over the edge but the slave was quick to lap up the few remaining drops. They were quickly lost from view in the crush of flesh but I already knew I was going to enjoy the evening. Even this crowd rarely witnesses such public displays of submission.

I gave up on the washroom. If it came to it, I would piss against the wall. It wouldn't be the first time this place had been baptized in this manner. With these lineups it was evident that I would be here all night, so I returned with a mug of Coke to where I had been standing. The slave was still on his knees, his cheek rest ing comfortably on his Master's boot.

"Wasn't as bad as I thought, " nodding back at the masses.

He just nodded a reply, his gaze lost on someone in the crawling circle of semi naked men.

The hunt continues. Even in this crowded place, I noticed the

subtle shift around our presence. By myself, I was given person-
al space and respectful elbowroom. But the three of us were
granted just that much more space. Respect in such a crowded
environment? Doubtful. Intimidation, maybe. Fear, more likely.
You could see that fear in their eyes also. The fear to let go. The
fear of themselves; wishing with every fiber of their being that
they had the courage to trade places with the slave and his dish.
There was some scoffing and laughing, probably to cover their
own insecurities, but recognizing themselves in that boy on the
floor. Wishing they could give into all that surrounded them. The
eyes never lie. Other looked with approval. Both Tops and bot-
toms understand. They had been there. Again, the eyes never
lie. Still others transferred their need into sexual energy, a close
substitute for the power exchange that could set their hunger
free. Satisfied for a while, but never complete. The hunger always
returns. Whatever the cause of our isolation, it made the place
bearable. Few seemed willing to encroach on our territory. Even
those jostled close by the crowd offered apologies.

"Excuse me, Sir."

"Sorry, Sir." Their glances quickly averted.

With difficulty under the volume of the music, we carried on a
conversation, reminiscing old acquaintances and old times, when
my friend finally stepped out of the crowd. We hugged and I
looked at him as I held him by the shoulders at arms length. He
had matured. It was time to let go. He had become my equal in
my absence. He was no longer the boy I had tutored and I was
proud of him, yet a little sad at the same time.

"You look great," I said, at a loss for the right words.

"You too, Sir." I couldn't tell if he said that out of old habits or old
Leather respect.

He turned, put his arm around his friend, and drew him into our
circle. Pride on his face, showing off his new boy.

"Sirs," was the boy said.

He was respectful. The education had been passed along to the
next generation. I smiled to myself as a vision of Kirk giving over
command of the Enterprise to Picard passed through my mind.
My chuckle only confused the boy.

"Glad you could be here," I said, "and welcome to the family."

He hesitated briefly but then shook my hand. He looked surprised at the lack of formality. I wondered what terrors had been conveyed about me. Introductions were made to the Master, and in turn the boy from Seattle. As our circle enlarged, so did the space around us. The conversation, and the evening drifted into the early hours of the morning. The atmosphere in the bar became more lewd as the 'witching hour' approached. More conducive to my growing raunchy mood.

"Must be all that sexuality in the air, that or the sugar rush from all the Cokes." I thought. I needed to piss badly, but it was too late to brave the line-ups now. Turning to the wall, I unbuttoned my leathers, and proceeded to relieve myself as unobtrusively as possible when a hand rested on my shoulder. I thought for a moment I had been caught by the bartender. The Master squeezed his hand, winked, and inclined his head in this slave's direction. Taking his cue, I drenched the T-shirt on the slave's back. Such sweet release. The Master opened his fly, and let go a golden stream also. By now the slave was saturated, lost in his own world between obedience and reward. His eyes lit up with excitement and understanding. This was his chosen station. The eyes never lie.

There were mixed reactions from those surrounding us. There is a big difference between in-role gratification and feeding a need through negative attention. For this slave, the act was one of supplication. For the Master, it was one of power exchange and possibly a reminder of the control placed within his trust. For myself, pure pleasure in sharing the gift.

The boy from Seattle expressed a look somewhere between disgust and excitement with undeniable intrigue. I wondered what else would engage his virile imagination this weekend. He seemed so young and full of wonder. I suddenly felt old. I turned to head for the bar. I needed another Coke.

I leaned on my elbows at the bar, staring at the television, but not seeing the movie that was playing. This was the back room of the AA, and the flicks here were not available back home. This was real porno, not that watered-down vanilla junk that customs allows into my country. But the pictures I was staring at were only in my mind. Snapshots of a young man challenging the sys-

tem in the only way he knew how: skiing. Not just respectful, family-oriented, Sunday racing camp skiing, but run-away-from-home-long-haired-rebellious-mongul-bashing skiing.

I had done my time in the organized kids racing camps and they taught me how to ski; very well too. I had raced all through university. At least for as long as I attended. I never did finish. After all, I was taking business administration and accounting. "Respectable, wear a tie," my mother said. And I had wanted to be an artist. Imagine such a thing! Also, this was still the Sixties, pre-love, do-your-own-thing counter-culture, and patriarchal families stilled ruled. So I left university, to work for an accounting firm. I lasted thirteen months, my lucky number. I got caught with ski magazines under my client's work. The firm frowned on billing clients for my personal reading time. Of course, I had missed the odd day when the snow was perfect also. Thus, I was fired. Subconsciously, I think I planned it because I didn't feel like I belonged there in the first place.

Those were good days. Taking all my life's aggressions out on a mountain. Too tired at night to think about the consequences of abandoning a career, never mind the condescending views taken by my parents. My first taste of anti-everything. And how I hated summer then. Skiing was Hollywood. Everyday was a good time, and all the people around me were there to have fun, relax, and enjoy life. Summer meant real work, real life, so I could do it again next winter. I did it next winter for fifteen years. It was glorious; free and broke.

It was civilized rebellion, being able to live on that mountain, knowing that I could get away with it because it was sports. Then, one September, on my way back to that mountain pilgrim age, I stopped in the city, found a phone booth, and dialed up the local 'Gay lines' information directory. I never made it to the mountain that year, or the one following, or the year after that. It was no longer necessary to lose myself in that world of sports and denial.

I smiled and looked down at the bar, both hands wrapped around my mug. "And look at me now, standing here in full leather, belonging." I continued my musing about the past.

I had parked my four-by-four in the lot, positioned to see the door of the gay bar. Every serious skier owned a four-wheel drive, it wasn't until several dates later that I discover how butch it was.

It took three tries to reach that door of the bar before I could open it to enter. I must have sat in the parking lot for an hour and a half before the first attempt, only to return to the truck. On my third attempt, I hesitated and opened the door. I stood there frozen, scared to death, immobilized and unable to move.

There was a doorman seated on a stool just inside. He looked in my direction, eyed me up and down, and squinted, "You a member?"

I reddened and stammered, "Ah, no..no..do I have to be?" I thought my heart was going to bounce right out of my mouth.

"Nah, just sign the book."

The doorman handed me an open loose-leaf book with a pen resting against the rings. I was shaking so badly that I dropped the pen, bent over to pick it up, and dropped the book also. I was aware of someone standing near the doorman who said "John, you are making the new guy nervous."

Was it that obvious? I almost bolted for the door. I was shaking violently as I signed a name. Not my own, of course; this was a gay bar for heavens sake, who knows where those names end up. As fast I could, I ordered a drink and headed for the nearest corner. Looking back on it now, everyone in that bar must have known I was there. I was new, frightened, and thrilled all at the same time.

I was distracted by the bartender returning my change. Chuckling at the memories that had flashed by in the time it took to pour a drink. I dropped a bill in the tip jar, retrieved my mug and headed back to the wall. I rejoined the group and leaned against the wall, my gaze surveying the available men. "Time to put all that seasoned experience to work," I thought.

It didn't take long. I spied a young man looking in my direction, questioning. I nodded. He lowered his eyes, and clasped his hands behind his back, snaking a glance back in my direction to see if I had noticed the gesture and I nodded again. Like I said, the eyes never lie. A small smile curled at the edge of his lips. My night was just beginning.

I have only one regret - that it took so long to discover this world of Leather. I think I always knew it was there, but I didn't acknowledge it until my late twenties. Coincidentally, my awareness heightened with the death of my mother. Whether I acted upon my desires because of her death or due to of the removal of an authoritarian figure, I do not know. I even considered the possibility that I was using SM to displace the anger I felt toward the family matriarch. I do know that I was suddenly free.

I recognized certain limitations of growing up in the Sixties and heeding my parents wishes. I had always wanted to be an artist, probably because I shared some small talent with (yes-here he is again) my uncle. But as was customary to the generation, my parents decided against my wishes. And that freedom manifested itself in several important ways. Things I have yet to place or explain, but I knew the relevance of that period changed my life. I remember the clarity of the events that changed things because of something that happened years later in San Francisco that helped put a lot of this in perspective chronologically.

San Francisco has changed many a man's life but I was already familiar with it's draw and comfortable, by that time, with myself. I was brought back to the memory of my awakening on a warm sunny day in the Castro. Several of us were sitting against the ledge of the Barracks Bar, just a few doors down from the Castro Theater. I think it is gone now because of the 'lets go look at the fags' attitude of the tourists. Anyway, I watched as several straight couples exited one of the those tourist busses and began timidly peeking in shop windows, obviously intimidated and probably not really sure who was watching who. "Were we on exhibit? Or were they?"

As the tour busses came and went through the afternoon, I began to notice certain reactions from the women. They were either totally comfortable and free in this all-gay, non-threatening environment, to totally paranoid. Those that were insecure about their presence, immediately grabbed hold of their husband's hand, arm or waist in a 'too-obvious' attempt to defend their territory. Ownership by decree of the ring on her finger. Their insecurities may not have been about themselves, but about their relationships. Maybe they sensed something threatening about their husbands or had self-doubts about their male companions. Remember, I said the eyes never lie. And it was evident in their eyes, watching some of those men step off the bus, that something 'clicked' about this place. Not so much an obvious reaction, but a feeling. More a sense that they were trapped in a world that they could now never escape, to explore the things that happened only in their imaginations. A flicker of recognition that maybe they had missed something, that this all looked too familiar. A lost world, suddenly discovered. And their wives sensed it also, and hung on all the more tightly, suffocating them, not out of fear for their well-being or safety, but out of the fear of losing him to 'us.'

And, like myself, some men probably did return, years later, because of that sea of awakening planted so accidentally. But to sit on that ledge, watching those straight men take it all in without any hint of redneck insecurities, in some small way saddened me. How long would some of them wait to be free? Would some ever overcome those forces in their lives that anchor them to a life they would rather not have accepted?

I have paid a high price for my freedom, in one sense or another, but I have never been happier or more self-aware. Like I said before, I wear my leathers with more purpose now.

Crack!

It must be close to a full moon. My sleep patterns have become erratic and restless. I sound like Lestat. I recognize that this body I inhabit has needs, it would just be a little more convenient to be able to control the timing. My inner clock hints at the impending, yet familiar; lust.

Lust is a wicked Master or Mistress. The timing is never appropriate or planned. A full moon is usually my nemesis, with a day or two before and after subjecting my hormones to that eternal pull of the tides against my soul. Werewolf - Vampire - Master, all legends, linked inexplicably to the sacrificial lust of the full moon.

I close my eyes, yearning to fulfill whatever basic needs are at hand, or in my hand, for that matter. Uncaring? To a point. But never out of control, edging toward fulfillment of whatever lies behind that veil of darkness that is relentlessly shrouded in varying degrees of lust. Uncaring, only in the search for release, but make no mistake, I care a great deal for those that share the journey. A shared quest. Often with only a glimpse of comprehension toward the pursuit of individual release. The ending unknown, yet predictably patterned. I also find that the need varies in intensity. Sometimes very little will satisfy the hunger. A simple shared touch. A foreign caress of my leathers. At other times, the need is so great that days are required to calm the dark tides.

I am older and wiser now - age being irrelevant - about the forces that drive my Leather. I can feel the need creeping into my soul, knowing that the time of the required act can be adjusted to fit a specific environment. Like snacks in the afternoon that hold you over until mealtime. Some small morsels of satisfaction that can be manipulated into a full contentment. Keeping the need alive until the right moment can either be found or maneuvered to accommodate an act of completeness. Such depth, such planning, such understanding of those needs comes only with experience. Lust.

I never tire of that primal urge. Even when taken by surprise, there is a spontaneous reaction to a visual image or thought that crosses my path with an instantaneous need to satisfy the urge. Unrelenting storms, winds of passion, pound wave after wave upon my soul, slowly subsiding, exhausting themselves on the rocky shores of my need. Philosophical? Maybe. But the adjectives don't carry the weight needed to explain the eruption of that primal urge and intense emotions. The label 'Leather' is too broad, yet incredibly accurate. It somehow encompasses all of this without having to say anything else. That solitary word says nothing - yet says everything.

I have come to realize that I do not approach problem solving within the parameters of normalcy, according to the AMA. Hopefully, no one I know fits those statistics. I would like to think that most folks are just a little more creative in their findings, right or wrong. In fact, I don't believe most Leatherfolk have even thought out their reason for including kink in their lives. It just is. It has always been there in one form or another. It doesn't always manifest itself in the overt forms of SM play, but is valid just the same, and rightfully so. After all, it would be pretty boring if we all dressed the same, played the same games, and approached out kink with assembly line precision. The missionary position suddenly comes to mind.

Bear in mind, however - and this is a big one - differences frighten people. But they excite some of us, too! On the whole though, most people circle cautiously until those differences become familiar. The problem with kink is that even though everyone has one, they don't always seem to be able to parallel theirs with someone else's: 'My kind is okay, yours is a little strange though.' And I am glad most folks approach it this way because distance provides security with one's kink. Again, if everyone was the same... The trick here is learning to respect others for their differences. I don't mean right-wing political differences, just those noticeable differences a little left of mine.

I started out by saying that I approach a problem from a different viewpoint. Comfort levels being what they are, most folks do not have the advantage, or disadvantage, of my view of the world: dark.

Here is a perfect example. My gallows humor lends a totally cynical view of a particular image. Probably the most politically incorrect thought is the one to cross my mind first, although it pops out of my mouth less often these days. I truly believe in standing up for the rights of others, especially if they are unable to stand up for themselves. But my 'how-could-you-say-such-a-thing' brand of humor is uniquely my own. Others seem to miss the point. Balance is a hard thing to learn. Blame it on a deficient childhood maybe, I don't know.

Our differences are our glue. They are what sticks us together. It is why we defend each other. Whether we understand each other's fetish or not, or whether we participate in some form of shared kink or not, it is our reason for assemblage. So what if your kink seems a little strange to me? Maybe mine seems a little off center to you also. Actually, I hope it does. It gives us something to discuss and share, especially in an intolerant society.

I very often hear 'under-your-breath' comments about certain individuals or lifestyle interpretations that seem just outside our norm. Odd using the word norm, as in normal, to describe kink in my redneck part of the country, never mind the AMA's version of normal. Anyway, the slashing we do to each other creates as much emotional turmoil as anything the outside world could do. I appreciate differences. They allow room for creativity, spontaneity, and interest in areas that I may not have had before. Dark humor may be way of dealing with a cynical world, but a tongue lasting, however haphazard or even consensual, scars and divides a community far worse than any physical beating.

Our ability to group our differences together for a more powerful voice has only touched the tip of the iceberg. There are so many people out there looking for a place to belong. We need to focus on our ability to reach out to those that are searching for any sign of acceptance. We need to make our differences a little more visible to those who are interested and cautiously offer the security of a **Safe, Sane and Consensual Environment** in which they may explore their kink. Then we will earn their respect by learning to respect each other.

Much has been borrowed from the Leather culture over the decades. Hollywood made the leather biker jacket a rebel trademark with the movie *Rebel Without a Cause*, largely in reaction to the gay bike clubs of the Fifties. They were post war misfits and misunderstood loners. The punk movement made most Old Guard Leathermen look respectable. But it's influence also changed the look and attitudes of a younger generation of Leathermen. MTV, heavy metal, and country music have also made the leather jacket, chaps, and motorcycle accessories acceptable street wear.

Musically sexualized leathers. Gosh, I wonder who could have influenced all that overt sexuality in the music industry? The music industry has had more influence than they know. I have seen high school kids with cock rings hanging off their epaulettes, totally unaware of the symbolism. Mad Max made leather accessible, flashy, but not honest in an Old Guard sense. And, watching the movie *Police Academy*, I peed myself laughing at the leather bar scene only because most of the people in the audience took it so seriously. A Leather bar is serious business, but even I can laugh at myself once in a while. Homophobia may be rampant, but leather phobia is even more so. Nothing reinforces the imagination more than the unknown. Much may have been borrowed from the Leather culture in satire, but leather has also borrowed much from our ancestors such as ritualism, tribalism, and rites of passage.

Crack!

I threw my jacket over my shoulder as I left the bar. The night was humid, sticky and warm, but I don't mind. It felt good, after all, it was snowing back home. I looked up at the night sky through the palm tress, pinpoints of light winked back. A shiver passed through my spine. Premonitions? Maybe. My mother used to say that someone had stepped over your grave when you shivered involuntarily. I won't be able to tell if someone does.

I was in Orlando, Florida, and the back patio of the Saloon Bar was crowded. Someone gently pushed their way by, excusing themselves as they passed. I had been so lost in the moment that I had not moved, blocking the entrance to the bar. I moved up the rail, threw one leg up and sat side-saddle over looking the crowd. It was so much nicer out here; free of the smoke and heat of the bar, a gentle breeze cooling the sweat on my neck above my vest.

As my eyes adjusted to the darkness, I could see forms moving about in the bushes at the edge of the crowd. The air was ripe with the urgency of those needs being fulfilled in the dark recesses of the fenced-in courtyard. More than once, I heard the sound of piss splashing against the paving stones. The conversation, as well as the music, was low, punctuated with the odd laugh, as befitting this open, free, and almost wild place. It was paradise. Well, at least to me. I was enjoying the nice warm weather and smelling the salt in the air. It was February with two feet of snow back home and I would be bundling up just to start the car. I shivered again. "Paradise."

My inner drive is always stronger in warmer climates and it was reaching gushing proportions, but I was in no hurry to find a release. I was waiting with sweet anticipation for the right moment; the right boy.

I slid off the rail and headed back inside for another drink, regretting the fact that I had brought along my jacket, although almost everyone else was wearing one. I pulled open the door, at the same instant, the bartender was shouldering his way out with a tray full of beer. The combination of my forward momentum and the unexpected release of the heavy door sent the bartender's shifting weight directly into a spin and disaster. The collision was unavoidable. I stood there drenched in beer and disbelief. The sudden silence was deafening. Just as suddenly, several hands extended to help. The crowd resumed its noisy exuberance as apologies were extended for both myself and the bartender. This wasn't exactly the scene I was looking for. The bartender made much fuss as he tried uselessly to mop some of the beer from my vest and chaps with a cloth. Most of the beer had hit me directly in the chest and had soaked down into my jeans.

"I-I-I'm sorry…Sir! Let me help. Here…let me wipe it off."

I smelled like a brewery.

"No. No. It's my fault. I shouldn't have pulled the door away from you like that," I said.

"At least let me clean your leathers up, or bring them back so I can clean them?" he asked.

"Yeah, yeah, I better go change." I hurriedly left the bar, almost as embarrassed as the bartender.

"Great!" I thought. "So much for the night. Good thing I brought other clothes."

It was a short walk through a mobile home park to the Parliament House motel. I stripped out of the wet clothes, threw them in the tub, and hopped onto the bed. I lay there wondering how to rescue the evening, knowing that I should just write this one off but not wanting to.

What was it he said? Something about cleaning my leathers, I think. It all happened so fast that it was tough to remember that small conversation. I looked at the clock. It was almost two A.M.

Maybe if I took the chaps over, he would at least be able to get the beer smell out. Then again, maybe I should just leave them - it adds flavor for the next boy. Some joke. I take care of my leathers. Naked, I padded into the bathroom, retrieved the chaps, and put them into a plastic bag. I slid into a pair of torn jeans, a T-shirt, and the wet boots. They were the only ones I had with me, so they'd have to do.

The crowd was thinning as I entered the bar. It was almost closing time. The bartender had his back to me, hands in the sink, as I set my package on the bar. He turned, grabbed an empty glass next to me, and said, "What can I getcha, bud?" without looking up. He dropped the empty glass in the sink, then looked up to see what I would order. Recognition set in and he lost all confidence.

"Hey, look I'm sorry about earlier, let me buy you a drink."

I didn't answer. Instead, I slid the bag across the bar in his direction, never losing eye contact.

He blinked, "What's this?"

"You said you'd clean them. So that's why I'm here...boy."

He lost it. Unsure what to do or how to answer, he just stood there knuckling the bar rag in his hands. "Uh...yes, Sir...I did ...didn't I ...uh, Sir." He was staring intently at the rag in his hands now. Someone rapped a glass on the circular bar behind him, trying to get his attention.

"Look after your customers" I said, "I'll wait."
He turned, and I wondered what was going through his mind. His hands were shaking a bit as he poured the drinks. When he finished, he returned with a mug of beer, and set it in front of me.

"I'm sorry, I don't indulge," I said as I pushed it aside, "but you can get me a coke."

Now he was more flustered than ever. I wasn't sure why I had bothered to returned to the bar or why I continued to hang around. I couldn't salvage the evening now and a little soap and water would easily clean up leathers. So why was I so determined to make this young man responsible for the accident? It was just as much my fault as his.

He politely placed a coke on the bar and, with a much practiced move, smacked the till open, flipped the lights, and turned down the music. The flash of the lights signaled closing time. Counting out the float as the till rang out its totals, he nodded and acknowledged familiar patrons leaving the bar.

"Hey guy! Time's up!" he shouted to a couple in the corner groping frantically, totally unaware of the time and the lights, urgently pursuing the night.

Finally, we were alone, as he scooped up glasses from around the bar and placed them in the dishwasher. Pulling a set of keys from the till, he locked both sets of doors, and plopped himself down on the stool next to mine. Rotating. With his back to the bar, he leaned back on his elbows, tilted his head back, and sighed, "What a night."

I was now as curious about him, as I was about my own motives for returning. I turned to study this young man. His look was easy, and casual. He was wearing a plaid sleeveless shirt, well worn, which somehow added to his comfortable manner and showed off his well developed arms. The shirt was open to his jeans which were also well used, revealing a dark patch of chest hair. He was rugged looking and I was enjoying the view, but I was still wasn't sure why I had come back.

I looked away and glanced about at the western paraphenalia hanging above the fireplace. A rope, bridle, branding iron, and saddle were draped over the open beam. All those years of growing up on the ranch flashed by. It would easily have made a bunkhouse on the ranch where I grew up. I looked in the young man's direction again, then back to the saddle on the rafter. Bingo! My disappointment with the evening turned full circle as scenarios flashed all over the place in my mind. I could imagine him standing on a bar stool suspended by his wrists from the stirrups of that saddle. Or spread-eagle against the fireplace strapped to the mantle with his feet tied to the outside of the iron grate within. Or stretched over a bar stood, all four limbs secured to the legs, with me holding the branding iron in my hand, menacingly. I smiled, "God, this was more fun that actually doing it. Well, almost." He broke the spell.

"I gotta get some sleep," he said as he reached for the plastic bag containing my chaps, "besides, the cleaning crew will be here any *minute." His reactions were too quick. His nervousness revealed some manner of indecision. Of what? I didn't know. The moment was shattered.*

I pushed myself away from the bar, rose, and hooked my thumbs into my pockets. I wasn't sure - did I let the moment slide? Was I just not reading this one right? No signals at all were forthcoming or was it just a case of nerves on his part? Of course, if he had been working here for any length of time, he knew how to mask everything. Everything but indecision. I still didn't know why I had returned. It was up to him. I knew I was in the mood to oblige but I needed more than that and he didn't seem to want to commit. He stood nervously in front of me.

"May I return these to you tomorrow, Sir?" he asked as we headed for the door.

"I would expect that. How's four o'clock? What time's your shift?"

"Not until ten, Sir. That would be fine, Sir."

"Good. Room 24 then," I replied, "Oh, and wear a jock-strap, you'll be needing it."

"Excuse me?"

"You heard me, boy," I said with a bit of an edge to my voice, testing his reactions.

"Yes, Sir, be glad to, Sir."

I stepped through the open door and, without looking back, crossed the parking lot. I could hear the keys locking the door as I stepped into the dark shadows of the night.

I suppose I have never really had the courage to look deeply into my bottoming experiences. Not because I was afraid of what I might find, but of what I might feel. Emotions are often difficult to assess. Especially your own. But the raw emotional responses to SM are so visceral that they become almost impossible to decipher without some guidance or interpretation as to their meaning. Hence, the Old Guard applications; learning by example, the things that can only be taught by doing. Things that were never written down but were passed along by the elders of our tribe. Absorbing the thoughts and consciousness of a culture that cannot be described, nevermind identified. The emotions that surface, sometimes including those from the past, require some form of guidance or channeling to be effective learning tools. Most often, the presence of an older Leatherman will stabilize or neutralize those fears and apprehensions that accompany such strong emotional releases. And, I don't for one minute think that older applies to chronology in terms of age, but in terms of knowledge about, not only our culture but also the human experience. As I have said before, many young men have acquired the skills necessary to guide others because of their understanding of past experiences.

Except for the similarities in the uniform of leather (and even that has subtle individual differences), the only 'cultural glue' is the intangible knowledge of SM. Much like the native cultures that existed for thousands of years, Leatherfolk share a verbal history that is rich with tradition. Tangible only in spirit, different with every telling, and different also by the perceptions and experiences of those conveying the message. Yet, the essence and heart of the message is so similar among communities separated by socio-geographic and socio-economic boundaries. Similar to all those ancient cultures that built some form of pyramid - different in style or interpretation, but still a pyramid just the same. Thus I learned, sometimes unknowingly, sometimes against my will, the lessons that were passed into my heart more than my hands. There may have been times I could not have identified the physical portions of the play as valuable emotional insights, but lumping all the years of experience together gave me, pun intended, a Master's Degree. Or at least a degree of understanding of the need shared by so many.

During my early years, I witnessed a Master lay a vicious flogging on two boys who were tied together, face to face. I remember thinking how cruel he was to have dealt such a beating and then just walk away ignoring their whimpers and lashed backs. What I could not have known, and a good lesson learned, was that the experience had been one of bonding for the two bottoms. The act had been measured and meted out to forge those emotional bonds required for support through other trying times when the boys may not have had the luxury of each other's company. But they could at least relate to the other's experience for emotional support at a later time.

Nothing I could have gleaned from the books and magazines available at the time could have replaced the very necessary experience of entering this community as a bottom. I mean bottom in terms of student, not necessarily submissive. The very act of learning balance between our SM play and the emotional comfort necessary to accommodate that play is one of time. And, for some, that time is longer than for others.

There are many Tops who are well read, who can talk the talk and even walk the walk, but the depth of knowledge is only as deep as the last article they happen across. And I don't say this to denigrate anyone - I wish I had the material that is now available when I was searching for more education. You can read all you want about rock climbing, fondle the rope, even touch the rock but, until you have stepped away from the edge of the precipice and trusted your knowledge and those minuscule tools that bind you to the cliff as Master, then the experience is only two-dimensional, not quite whole. Black and white versus Technicolor. Watch and learn, experience then share your conclusions with someone in a position of trust. Ask your bottom or Top about the experiences you have shared, whether in the past or as recent as moments ago. Discover that balance is not a measured thing. Notice, too, that SM is not equal in measurement to the experience required. By that I mean, interpret the experience correctly; there does not have to be intense pain to acknowledge the experience or scene and call it SM. Circumstances and mood rule the events. Often, a couple of well placed words or a simple touch will offset hours of play, but sometimes, the opposite is true. An off gesture or comment may take time to equalize roles or centralize attitudes.

Crack!

We were standing in the open window of the Barracks Bar on Castro Street. Four of us; two Tops and our boys. As usual, the bar was packed and yet, we had managed to secure some personal space within which to talk and still watch the crowd pass by on the street. As crowded as the bar was, one of the patrons managed to seat himself close to us near the window ledge. Discussions evolved and revolved around various topics and the man seated next to us seemed to be paying no attention - he only occasionally glanced in our direction although, he was close enough to be privy to our chat.

As the evening wore on, the bar crowd thinned a bit, allowing for more elbow room. The man on the ledge became more intent on our group and I noticed his attention being drawn to the chain and collars that the boys wore which were padlocked. Conversation drifted to the crowd outside and the amount of leather visible on the street. Suddenly, the man was on his feet, poking a finger into my chest.

"You out-of-towner's, you think you are so tough, so butch, well,

I have lived here for sixteen years - this is my playground - you have a lot to learn," he slurred, and the smell of beer wafted around him.

Mid-sentence, my boy was on his feet adopting a defensive position, wedging his way between us and the verbal assault continued. I was momentarily stunned by the vehemence. He wavered a moment, looking almost as surprised as we did at the outburst, then, inexplicably, staggered for the exit. I patted my boy on the shoulder, relaying both thanks and comfort with his actions, as he dutifully seated himself again.

Whatever revelry had been attained by our small party was lost and we soon dissipated into the cool evening, lost in our thoughts as we headed back to our rooms. I was baffled by the event. Most vanilla folk misunderstand us at the best of times, but the actions of that bar patron were not to be easily passed off. What was it that bothered me? I usually let stronger comments than his bounce off my leather armor. What had the obviously intoxicated fellow meant? Was his outburst a social commentary on our leathers? Did he consider us rebels not willing to fit into his view of the world? Was he an experienced player and upset that we had failed to recognize him? After mulling over the event, I began to see a far different pattern. I began to see an individual so insecure and lonely that his only recourse was to lash out in frustration. An individual that could not fathom a culture that so visibly showed affection and support for each other as a family.

I began to speculate. Here was a man who had lived in Mecca for sixteen years, sitting in a bar alone on a Saturday night; no friends to mingle with. He was probably depressed, lonely, and desperate for the camraderie and support that so many of us take for granted. I began to almost feel sorry for him. Again, I wondered, had he had an unpleasant experience at the hands of a Leatherman? A broken relationship maybe, or a wrong turn personally? Or had he lost so many acquaintances to the plague that his perspective of the gifts of life shifted radically into depression? I gave up. I would never know what his thoughts, however incoherent, were.

But I was changed by that moment somehow because, in a lot of ways, he was right. Those words at face value, "you have a lot to learn," could not have been spoken at a better time. It took my ego down a few notches and I realized over the next few days just how much I did not know about my tribe or my community. A few drunken words tossed about in anger caused me to plant my feet firmly with the knowledge that I am a proud Leatherman pursuing the lessons of my elders.

This is a community that is constantly evolving, growing, and changing. It's basic values may remain constant, but the energy, new ideas, and fresh look help balance it's ideals and philosophies with every new experience. At least I enjoy doing the homework.

Crack!

I held my breath. Wrong. I should have been breathing to let the oxygen flow through my veins. At least that is what my brain told me. But my nerves and a small bit of fear just wouldn't let me follow my own intuition. How many times I had pierced someone with all that professional confidence and ease, conveying trust. If I could just trust my own advice.

My eyes crossed as I watched the two gloved hands approaching my nostrils. One held an enormous hollow needle, the other a cork. In actuality, the needle was only a fourteen gauge but it looked to be the size of a pen at that close range. I should have kept my eyes shut like he said.

This wasn't the first time Al and I had pierced each other and we had discussed this one many times before actually committing to the act.

His little fingers reached my nose first, cautiously twisting the needle and cork away from me, searching for the triangle separating the cartilage of my septum.

"This could be difficult," I said, "I have had facial reconstruction from a motorcycle accident."

"Hold still!" was all he said, "now, take a breath and let it out slowly."

I heard the needle more than felt it. I could have sworn it passed through an inch of cartilage, not just simple flesh. Tears welled in my eyes involuntarily, and one rolled freely down my cheek. The retainer slid easily into place next, but for days I felt like I had a railroad spike stuck through my nose. I was proud of my new *acquisition and was smiling, almost giddy, as tears rolled down my cheeks. I thought, "Some tough Top I was. Take it - yeah, sure!"*

I remember waking in the middle of the night after receiving that piercing, tears on my cheeks because I had accidentally rolled over in my sleep onto the new piercing at the tip of my nose. I sat up, wide awake, blinking because the healing time was still in progress and the pressure, as light as a feather pillow, still had the ability to shock me out of a deep slumber. I swear, up-gauging is more painful than receiving the piercing in the first place.

How many times had Al and I helped each other change gauges because it was just a little too much to push through to the next sized gauge ourselves?

I watched the new ring slide through - quickly, of course - and then waiting with my toes curled in my boots for the sensations to signal my brain. Wimp. How did I ever get through all those years as a bottom? Although, I did change my nipple rings myself - at work no less! Up-gauging from eight to six. They had arrived in the mail and, after a quick soak in peroxide, I pushed - more like rammed - one through at a time. Then, clutching the edge of my desk, I waited for the inevitable burst of light that signaled the expanding scar tissue after each insertion.

No one guessed why I was in a good humor as I walked around the office all day with a glazed look in my eyes. I wondered what everyone would say if they could see what was under my shirt. The rings and tattoos, held in pride and in secret from suburbia. Keeping them insulated and protected not from any fear of their visibility, but because I just don't want to take the time to explain, even in the vaguest term, my life or my needs.

Crack!

Several onlookers witnessed the dark, sensual whipping dance. We were at a dungeon party in Portland. The scene was special and I could sense an elusive connection with my bottom that rarely happens. We both knew it. A semi-circle formed around us, the whip defining personal space. The scene seemed to last an eternity, but it was all of maybe 30 minutes of magic ritual. My whip sung across her back. Yes. Her. I am an equal opportunity offender. Many people are curious, but few see that dark dance

82

with my whip. And those that can, provide a connection that is so pure and so rare that gender becomes irrelevant.

I teach about whips in many workshops. Whip play changes you and your perceptions of both the scene and the relationships that evolve around it. Little things, nothing tangible, but you become different somehow. I recall reading Dune and relating to the chemical that turned people's eyes blue. In relation to SM, as long as those people did not ingest that chemical, they would go on living; but having once tasted it, they had to keep up a steady diet or die. Metaphorically, my whips have done the same to me. I have played in other worlds in and around SM for years, but upon experiencing the whip, I was forever changed. Not floggers; whips. Single tails. Snakes with a very addictive bite.

"Sir, are you bi?" asked the young man with a collar who had approached me after the scene. "My Sir would like to ask about the whips."

"Nope. I am sure enough gay. I like dick." Besides, I thought, what would practicing my trade have to do with my orientation? I have bottomed to some very skilled Tops of many persuasions. That is, not to say that I am not into a little experimenting. I am secure enough with myself to explore all kinds of possibilities. If I get turned on doing a scene with a lesbian or a straight woman, what is the harm in exploring those consensual possibilities? I laugh as I remember being negotiated as a piece of rubber once, and then strapped to a lesbian so that she could butt-fuck her bottom using me as a substitute dildo. When I get the opportunity to share an experience, gender quickly fades into the black recesses of the dungeon and those that witness such exchanges are also changed.

It is amazing to me how many people are drawn to the sound of a whip. That crack that splits the sound barrier. The atmosphere that the sound creates at a dungeon party becomes sexually charged and intense. It's in the eyes and the eyes never lie.

My favorite boy says that the whip is his life line. He also calls it "lightning on a sunny day". I feel the balance during a scene; a tenderness that belies the visual of that whip slicing the air and cracking just above the back, caressing the back just slightly stronger than a kiss. It is hidden beneath the power and the sound and delivering those little welts of trust and need, commu-

*nicating in ways neither of us will ever be able to explain or dupli-
cate with any satisfaction. However, we will both search to repeat
such a magic moment, knowing full well that each time is different, special and so unprecedented that the search is in vain. For
me that is what makes these encounters so philosophical and
unique. The ability to share beyond known boundaries. A close-
ness and commitment that builds friendships and families with no
expectations, just a willingness to share and be secure enough to
know that the bonds forged through pain are their own metaphysical, sensual, and fulfilling rewards.*

I have no idea where the following piece came from but I find it appropriate to mention. The author is unknown. This is not meant as a copyright
infringement, but to honor it.

The Gift and the Giver, the Rebel, the Thief, and the Stranger and His Glue.

The Giver was alone and the Gift unused; the Giver felt lonely
and sought to find someone worthy of the Gift.

The Rebel came along and saw the Gift the Giver possessed and
desired the Gift for himself. Rather than ask the Giver for the Gift,
or ask what the Giver wanted for the Gift, the Rebel decided that
social rules did not apply to him and simply said, "Give me the
Gift."

The Giver knew that the Gift was fragile and would be destroyed
if mistreated and did not trust the Rebel for how many of those
who are impolite are also delicate? But the Giver did not wish to
offend and so said to the Rebel, "I am sorry, but this Gift is for
someone else."

The Rebel grew angry and blustered, "But I deserve the Gift. I
am special and I deserve that things be given to me."

The Giver, glad to have trusted his first instinct, merely repeated,
"I am sorry but this Gift is for someone else."

And the Rebel, still complaining, went his way.

The Giver sat under a willow tree contemplating the Gift and wondering about the qualities needed to really appreciate the Gift. As she was sitting there, the sun and the breeze and the sound of the creek below lulled her into a doze.

The Thief, who had overheard the Rebel and Giver, was waiting for just this moment. Dashing out from behind a nearby bush, he made a grab for the Gift; grasping it, he started to run away.

The Giver, however, was awakened by this and reached out to stop the Thief. "Give that back!" cried the Giver. "It is not yours! You have no right!" So saying, she reached out, trying to retrieve the Gift.

The Thief said, "I do not care if it was not mine. I have possession of it so it is now my property." And so saying, he pulled again at the Gift, hoping to wrench it from the Giver.

In the ensuing struggle, the Gift was fouled, battered, and broken. The Thief, deciding he did not want a damaged Gift, finally let go and said, "You keep it, it is now worthless."

The Giver cried at the state of the Gift which she had hoped to find someone worthy of; it was dirty, pieces were missing and scattered in the grass around her, and the intact parts were bent and dented. She began to believe the Thief's assessment of the Gift; perhaps it no longer mattered who it belonged to, worthless as it was.

But then she noticed that her tears made clean streaks on the Gift as they fell, and she thought that perhaps if some of it could be cleaned, all of it could; perhaps she could make her Gift have worth once again. She took the Gift and it's broken pieces to the creek where she began to wash them.

The Gift was easy to clean, but in trying to wash the pieces that had been broken from it, the Giver lost one. She began to lose hope again. Yet she was still determined to try to repair the Gift.

Hours passed as she fit the pieces back together where they would stay. Some pieces she could not make stay, however.

From behind her, a voice, "Perhaps this Glue could help you mend your Gift." She turned to see a Stranger holding a small tube of Glue. She took the Glue and thanked the Stranger, then finished her Gift with the Stranger's Glue.

When she turned to the give the Glue back to the Stranger, he was gone. She thought to herself that his Stranger had thought her Gift worthy enough to donate his Glue and not even demand payment, nor even ask for the Glue to be returned. Perhaps her Gift had worth after all.

And as she sat and contemplated her Gift, she realized that the Stranger was the type of person who would neither ask nor demand a Gift, not would he take it, but rather, he would give. She thought to herself that the Stranger was a Giver too. And who better to appreciate a Gift but a Giver?

So, she sought out the Stranger and when she found him, she tried to return the Glue to him. He thanked her but said that she should keep the Glue, in case the Gift should break again.

And the Giver said. "In that case, you should accept the Glue, for I wish to give the Gift to you." And, so saying, she placed the Gift in the Stranger's hands.

The Stranger looked at the Gift and said, "This is too precious. I do not know if I can take care of the Gift." The Giver said, "I believe that you can. I will stay with you and help you care for the Gift when you falter."

So, the stranger and Giver took the Gift together, sharing it, and holding it as an example for all to see.

I believe that the Gift could be interpreted in many ways but I will try to explain what it means to me.

If you are offering a Gift of your pain and your vulnerabilities to someone you trust only to have those areas that one holds so private cruelly mistreated, then extending that trust a second time becomes near impossible. Rejection is the harshest Master. The search for acceptance can become almost maddening in it's intensity and it's need. One becomes wary and mistrustful. After all, why risk such personal humiliation? And, at what point do you begin to trust again, and how do you recognize a safe place in which to deposit that trust? Yet, it is that act of robbery that makes most of us worldly or street smart, enabling us to parcel out portions of ourselves to individuals who gain our trust.

We do learn to measure that which is needed or extended by body language. It is in the eyes. Dare I suggest that when the least is expected, the most is gained? Maybe I should rephrase that to say that when something you hold precious is extended for view, without judgment, then the possibility to forge bonds of understanding is available. Even in the very basic attraction that may require no verbal contact, the chance of rejection is overturned by merely extending an interest. SM is definitely one of those areas of vulnerability. The fear of exposure, not on your terms, may send most into hiding. I know many people who have placed years of pre-imagined scenes at risk of rejection by unknowingly placing or misplacing their trust. Erotically driven fantasies most often go awry and expectations remain unfulfilled.

Novices are especially at risk. With the volume of one handed fiction available, many have retreated into their closets through misunderstandings or purposeful cruelty at the hands of self-styled players. Very few summon the courage to venture out again, their needs overriding their fears. But imagine the elation and feeling of salvation that one achieves when the time, the mood, and the connection is made. They finally realize their self-worth and suddenly find family, community, and a sense of belonging.

Three words have becomes the motto of Leatherfolk worldwide. They are **SAFE, SANE, and CONSENSUAL**. As we cling to the refuge of hope in a sea of grief called **AIDS**, those three words are more than a motto, they have become a life line. Many discussions arise at the mention of those three words because they represent a wide view of interpretations. Some usually orient toward medical safety but expand into emotional triggers and physical well being of the players involved. I think that emotional safety is a point that needs to be stressed more in workshops and discussions. Not that the others are not important, but they are more easily and thoroughly discussed.

If the players involved have not adequately covered some of the ground rules of conduct, then their play may be treading on thin ice unknowingly. Certain words may trigger emotions from a past that may not be too pleasant or could be down right horrific. Nothing is more frightening than having a play partner recede into emotional panic without any knowledge of the trigger. Body motions, certain circumstances, lighting or lack of it, may all play in factoring problems. A few honest exchanges at the beginning of an encounter may make the difference.

Common sense dictates that if you are uncomfortable in certain situations, then avoid them or make them known to your partner. Filling out a questionnaire may sometimes be easier than direct conversation.

Unfortunately, some people feel that discussing certain issues is viewed as a weakness rather than a practical solution. Many players seem to have no problem role playing and asking about a condom or rubber gloves within the play, but to ask about a word or specific actions containing unpleasant memories seems somehow inappropriate.

Stopping in the middle of play to ask a person not to use a word in no way detracts from the reality of the experience. After all, the idea is to enjoy the experience, not to perpetuate feelings of guilt or self-humiliation. If the play is being used to justify feelings of inadequacy then you shouldn't be looking for a Leather experience, you should be looking for a psychiatrist. Consent and sanity are more easily discussed in both a workshop situation and as ground rules for a period of play.

A problem I consistently come across is the fear of rejection or the feeling of having to consent to an activity a person is unsure of or does not enjoy, in order to prove themselves. You do not have to do anything you do not wish to do. You have the right to direct the play to your liking, or just say no. Easier said than done, I know, but a lack of playmates is no reason to jeopardize your well being. I have been told time and again that there are not enough good Tops around so a bottom feels he has to oblige in order to have an experience. Most Tops became good players by being versatile and adapting to the needs of BOTH players. Consent may be given verbally, but body language never lies, and a good Top will usually be able to read the information transmitted.

This is where I question the sanity of some player's use of drugs and alcohol. Perceptions of play and thresholds slide with the use of both because they influence judgment and reality. Ask questions. Find out if your partner has much, if any, experience in the activity you are interested in. If not, discuss why the activity appeals to you and ask questions of someone who is familiar with that activity. Ignorance is no excuse for an accident. Besides, paramedic fantasies can be fun and, if you are afraid of calling 911, fear not, they have seen it all.

No two people in a room are going to agree on the description of the words, safe, sane, and consensual. Negotiation is the key to an exciting experience, and the more you know about the motives of the play, the more rich the experience becomes. Every scene should end satisfactorily and, if not, try to discuss where things went stale or perhaps where miscalculations crept in. Remember, masturbation fantasies rarely endure in reality. You are responsible for your own rewards. We all look for the same things; the comfort of body contact, reassurance of emotional support, and the joy of achieving our orgasms or expectations. It is very difficult to open up and bare your soul, but starting off slow and discussing an evening's events will help build the excitement of future encounters.

To understand Leatherfolk, one has to understand the social order to which the lifestyle is applied. The empowerment that accompanies the affirmation of the Leather lifestyle has been compared to a second coming-out. The rigidity, respect, and unspoken code of ethics that exist at the core of all Leather organizations are built around the need for structural self-preservation. Probably the most important thing I have learned from the travels and experiences of the North American Leather Community is the politics of shock value. As Leatherfolk, we are a visible, viable part of a larger community which has demonstrated time and again the importance of diversity.

There is a fine line between 'consent with an audience' and an 'in your face' attitude. Both are useful political tools that work for us as well as against us. Leatherfolk have been expounding the difference between consent and abuse for years. To those in the Leather community, there is trust, consent, and understanding of the nuances of the lifestyle. To the unaware and uneducated, public play is often seen in a very negative light.

Politics? The dimmer the light, the more condemnation. Tolerance is a very personal thing and acceptance levels can vary, even among our own. The acceptance we strive for in the large community should not be judged by the actions of a singular negative (or perceived negative) incident. First impressions hold the most attention. Our community is a microcosm of the real world and, as such, there are applicable social problems.

Here are some of my personal views on code, or ethics:

- Thou shalt respect the privacy of others.

- Thou shalt not spread vicious gossip. Gossip creates alienation and no one trusts gossip.

- Thou shalt be of good humor. Common sense should tell you that a bad mood reflects on everyone in a social setting. There is no need for stress in our social escapes.

- Thou shalt be of moral support.

- Thou shalt speak out. Constructive criticism is important, and membership to this community has its responsibilities.

- Thou shalt leave prejudices at home. I am always amazed at the gay community's response to racial/gender diversity and that bigotry is tolerated by our own minority.

- Thou shalt not attract scornful attention or bring dishonor upon oneself or members of the community.

- Thou shalt be always conscious of the inherent dignity of Leatherfolk. After all, it takes courage to walk into a social setting in leather and the statement presented can be a visible and/or visceral trigger to emotional responses.

The above 'commandments' were the result of many discussions with a couple of dear friends. One is long gone now, but the memory of his participation in my 'education' carries much weight and value. And to the other, I offer my continued friendship. Thanks Dwight and Stephen.

Crack!

I asked all the wrong questions. Actually, I wasn't supposed to ask any of the questions; he was. This was supposed to be an interview of the lifestyle. Instead, it became a very revealing exchange, mostly self-incriminating on his part. I challenged why he kept coming back to question certain activities within my culture.

I am aware that people are curious about the dark and kinky side of sex. Like those old horror movies - scare me to death, then scare me again. Especially since (lately, at least) SM innuendo can be viewed on daytime TV and talk shows, not to mention the fashion industry's fascination with the look. The question was, who was interviewing whom?

He had done some homework. He knew, for instance, that there was a visual code - left and right symbolism. Although he had the sides misinterpreted, he understood their applications. He couldn't have known what I was thinking. I knew why he was here. There was so much he wanted to know that couldn't have been applied to a simple interview. An interview designed for a local alternative paper. I knew that he had a grasp of the connection between what represented the fantasies that maneuvered ellipti-

cally around his mind. This was the safest way for him to explore that dark mystery without risk of exposing his own interests. Or so he thought.

I shook my head. Had I become so intuitive that this boy was so much like an unopened book? He was new and fresh and so full of wonder which he disguised as hypothetical questions in the interest of his readership. Once again, I felt like Lestat. Do I take him where he really wants to go or just place him on that carousel of endless questions? I held myself in check but I wanted him. I knew he was afraid but that made it even more exciting. I could feel the erotic need rising within me. I became distant with my next few answers and started to daydream, allowing my predatory fantasies to feed.

He must have sensed the change because he put down his pad of questions and turned off the recorder. The sound of the pad striking the table snapped me back to reality. He looked like a deer in the headlights, unwilling to move, but terrified of the weight bearing down on him. I smiled. It broke the spell but not his interest. The interview was over but he would be back. Maybe next time.

At what point I became aware that I was a Leatherman escapes me. I do know that it was long before I actively pursued the leather look. It had to be, because if I was comfortable in that attire, then I had obviously made some commitment to the need for a visual statement. I identified with an idea more than a conscious attachment to a group of individuals. I think that the greatest impact for me was that the leather look existed at all. Until that point, the only images available to my new found sexuality were of effeminate men wearing dresses and wigs and the Hollywood evil associated with those kind of people.

The role model that was Hollywood was definitely nothing to aspire to. Don't get me wrong, I have nothing but admiration for the 'drag' community; I think it takes a lot of balls to willingly and publicly transform and impersonate the opposite gender. But it came as a welcome surprise to me that gay could also be defined in the masculine. And such a discovery was a quantum leap from the school yard defamation that accompanied the term 'fag'. Real men who loved each other. It was always there, even in public, but somehow I had missed the billboard advertising.

My whole world changed. In one stroke of thought, all the pieces fell together and I consciously purchased a pair of chaps. Knowing what I know now, I hadn't even earned them. Well, sort of. I had earned them simply by becoming aware of my needs, just not in the Old Guard sense. I regret that, too. It might have been more special to have earned rather than acquire them. Again, at the time, I was not even aware of such men. They were only pictures in magazines. Until Halloween of that same year, I was not even aware so many people owned leathers. I got to know a few socially but was to afraid to ask any real questions.

About eight of us would phone each other once a month and say, "Wear your leathers tonight," so as not to feel awkward at the bar alone. It was a powerful image to watch the crowd separate when we walked in. We could go anywhere in the bar we wished and space was made for us. They feared us. We were dangerous and we knew it but in reality, we knew nothing at all. We were still so afraid to go out alone in our leathers. Time and knowledge conquered. We stumbled across the odd article that was non-fiction and learned what the 'look' meant and the difference between erotic novels and the serious side of leather. We knew how hot it was to be dressed in leather, but we didn't know what to do with it once the feeling was in motion.

Before I came out to Leather, I tricked with a man who became one of my best friends. At the time, we looked in his closet and it was half full of leather. I was surprised because I hadn't seen him out in it and he explained that he only wore it out of town as, "No one here would understand." He dressed me in a few pieces, placed me in front of the mirror, and told me how good I looked. I liked who I saw, but I had no clue how to handle that man in the mirror. I was self-conscious but aroused. And the man who dressed me up was on his knees. Silly me, I got undressed. Had I only known.

When I left that evening, he gave me a pocket book called The Leatherman's Handbook. I took it home and immediately forgot about it until he asked for it back. I had to go rummaging for it and, upon rescuing it, wondered why it had been so important. Why had he seemed irritated that I had not returned it? It was battered, pages earmarked so often the corners were missing, and the cover could hardly be read it had so many folds in it. I saw it as just an old book until I glanced inside and became totally mesmerized. I returned that book a few days later. I purchased an armband, wrapped it about the book, gift wrapped the package, and delivered it. When he answered the door, he knew. I was changed and our friendship grew from there.

I have owned a half dozen of the books since. I can't seem to keep them. I give them away to the needy. I also have one mounted in a framed case, signed by Larry Townsend. It is a treasure and precious to me.

I knew who I was before I read that book but I was unable to put it in to words or thought patterns that resembled such a process. The chaps I had purchased were, unknowingly, only the tip of the iceberg; the only expression I was capable of at the time. I was not so much naïve as unsure of where to look or, I suppose, what to look for. So it is no accident that I reach out and make myself available for questions and ridicule from a larger community that lacks understanding. The reward is watching the lights go on for someone in the crowd at the realization that this, too, is what they have been drawn to.

Honor has such depth for such a simple word. It is extremely complicated and intangible. It cannot be bought or sold, it must be earned. It cannot be given, it must be bestowed. A single thing which, in its simplicity, can only be acknowledged through the integrity of the owner. It stands alone, yet it is as visible and bright on the bearer as armor. Honor is worn with pride, not arrogance, and everyone recognizes it, though no one I know can define it. "Good personal character," the dictionary says, "Respect." But it is more than that. It is sometimes so subtle that it often escapes those who come across it.

Most Leatherfolk who have endured any time in the community carry themselves with the dignity and honor that is inherent to the territory; often times they do not even know they possess it. Not to denigrate anyone, but they have earned it so slowly that it has attached itself to them over time. Some of those to whom we owe the greatest respect stand last in the crowd. Not because of any wish to be anonymous, but due to security in their standing and observing, rather than posturing. They are strong yet not arrogant; they may stand alone, but they are not lonely. They are comfortable with the mantel because they have settled those questions of orientation and need, then settled into kink as a way of life.

Crack!

He stood there for a long time against the rail of the bar. His hair was gray and his beard was salt and pepper, and neatly trimmed. He was solidly built behind the leather vest with an icy stare that melted when he smiled.

I was new to all this. I hugged the far wall more out of fear than anything else, trying hard to be anonymous. I nursed a Coke and watched the pool table separating us in the haze and smoke of the bar. The two men playing pool were either oblivious of me or, more likely, just dismissed me as a 'wanna-be'. I was the only man in the bar without any leather.

The younger of the two had on chaps, very worn jeans, and no shirt. He was slim but toned. I don't remember what the other fellow was wearing except for his boots, (I swore that was the first thing I would buy), and his pants were tucked into those boots. They were engineer's boots, almost knee high, with two buckles at the top of the calf.

I noticed that the gray haired guy had not moved but the shirtless young man playing pool was doing everything he could to attract the older gentleman's attention. It was almost embarrassing, even for me. I may have been new to this, but even I thought he was trying too hard to be recognized. The young man lined up a shot on the table, mis-cued, and sent the cue ball bouncing off of the table over his cue hand. As he pivoted to recover the ball mid-flight, his cue swung in the direction of the older Leatherman leaning on the rail of the bar. Like slow motion, I could see the arc of the cue impacting its inevitable target.

I was so focused on the moment that the haze of the bar disappeared and I felt like I was standing beside the man at the bar. With the slightest movement, his hand intercepted the swing of that cue and froze it in the midair, just inches from his cheek. So startled was the young man, that he completely released the cue, and took a step back. The expression on the older man's face never changed but his eyes grew hard. He took two steps away from the bar and placed the cue in the wall rack.

The shirtless boy stood there baffled and unsure but the look he received spoke volumes. He knew that he had crossed some invisible line, but didn't know what to do now. Should he speak? Nod? He was lost, out of his league, and he knew it. Slowly, he turned back to the table, replaced the cue ball, and disappeared into the crowd. His partner shrugged, reached for the rack, and began sorting the balls for a new game and the next player.

I doubt anyone else in that bar even noticed, but I couldn't take my eyes off that Leatherman. In fact, he was the subject of many fantasies over the next few weeks. I may not have understood the exchange at the time, but I was aware of the attitude that was projected; the self-confidence and dignity with which he carried himself. I watched him for the rest of the evening. It wasn't the near miss with the young man that impressed me, it was the man's body language and the way in which I perceived him. His body language spoke of security and strength.

I never saw him again, but I owe him. Watching his interaction, almost fatherly, with the few men who spoke to him throughout the evening, taught me much about respect and honor. I'll never forget him. We learn so much of our culture through observing other Leatherfolk and the impact is almost incalculable. We unconsciously draw so much information with the use of non-verbal communication that it is no wonder the leather takes on the perception of armor. So much is carried with it and projected by it that we stand apart, not only from the larger gay population, but also from our own kinky family. We are separate individuals, yet part of the larger recognition.

Crack!

I bit my cheek. I couldn't help it. My nose started to run and I tried squinting, but nothing helped. "This is it, " I thought, "I am going to laugh out loud." I was helpless and at the mercy of my Top. There I was, bound in Saran-Wrap, supported only by a beam that had been purposely mounted in the center of the dungeon. I was secured to a wooden pole with only a thin layer of plastic film separating me from my Top. He stood in a jock-strap, boots and armbands, holding a blow dryer, like some nightmare in a hair salon. It was too much to bear! I knew I would regret the outburst, but I just couldn't control it. I should have used my safe word instead. Now, I have played with a ton of ingenious toys in the dungeon, but this was so unexpected. A light moment - that was about to turn serious.

He didn't say a word, just smiled along with me, humoring me. I felt a wave of warm air wash over me, I was afraid to laugh again, but did steal a look to see if he was holding a comb in the other hand. Warren Beatty flashed through my mind along with scenes from the movie Shampoo.

The wrap was shrinking. Shrink-wrap, not saran-wrap. It was then that the severity of my predicament settled in and the realization slowly crept up my spine.

As the blow dryer slowly warmed the plastic film, I began to sweat. Lightly at first, then profusely. He started at my thighs; it was tight, but not unbearable.

I'll save your cock and balls for later," he said sadistically. I like that in a Top.

He worked his way up my abdomen, slowly creating a girdle effect.. It was tightening… squeezing… maneuvering around me; behind the post, I could feel the shrink-wrap increase pressure on my forearms and wrists.

"So what happens when I lose circulation, or should I be more concerned about losing consciousness?" I thought. "Be calm. Think calm. Don't panic. Breathe."

It was good advice to myself but totally ineffectual. As the wrap contracted, I heard two popping /tear sounds emanate from my chest. I was relieved to look down and see that it wasn't anything I owned, physically that is. Rather, the beer bottle caps that had been placed against my nipples, smooth side to flesh, had burst through the plastic with their serrated edges. Two perfect little thumb-like nipples stuck out from the holes in the wrap, the nipple rings bouncing almost straight out as the pressure extended around the protruding flesh. They were like little volcanoes of fire. I took another breath and found that it wasn't as deep as the previous. And the next was more shallow yet. Oxygen deprivation. It was wild. Little stars were forming at the edge of my sight.

My peripheral vision receded. I was aware of an erection. My balls were constricted and the euphoria was magnificent. Someone was turning down the lights. The candles on the wall were awfully bright and then they started winking out, one by one, then peaceful darkness.

"Now what? I don't want to wake up yet; quit stroking my face! Well, maybe…I am thirsty. What is that lump under my side, and why can't I roll over? And why am I wet?"

Everything flooded back. What a rush! I was laying across his lap. He sat cross-legged on the floor with his boots digging into my side. My chest was wrapped in a towel and my pubic hair was matted. A bundle of wrinkled plastic wrap filled my vision. I closed my eyes again, happy and comfortable within his grasp. His touch was secure, reassuring and I felt more alive than ever. I don't know how close to not being alive I had been.

I trusted him totally and was so grateful. His fingers were exploring and his need grew against my back. I was his and wanted to *please; to know his release and his satisfaction. The heat of the room became stifling and the darkness comforting as he snuffed out the candles to leave only one.*

One of the dichotomies surrounding Leatherfolk is the tenderness and understanding of the human spirit that underlies all that is visual, encompassing a culture. It is terribly ironic that men and women can wield such incredible power within their own souls, sheltered within an exterior of hardened steel like a warm and cozy brick house buffeted by winter storms. "Insignificant and yet, supreme." I heard that somewhere and it fit.

We are considered a masquerade, yet we are not masking anything at all. Our symbolism and outward signals are so necessary to survival and recognition of the culture. There is a reason black has been a color of power of centuries. From pagan priests to royalty, from ancient nighttime rituals to present nighttime rituals, and from the need to melt into the night to the power from blending with the night. In some ways, the lights are kinder at night. Nothing is a harsh as the midday sun. In the bright light of day, too much is revealed. A full moon tugs at those ancient tides of the soul.

A little sappy maybe, but ask anyone connected to a hospital emergency ward how a full moon effects the tourists. And how, at any time of the month, it allows those emotions that require comforting to rise to the surface. Tenderness is protected from the night in black leather. It may well be buried under all that visual danger, that bravado, but its there just the same. There is nothing hard about these folks. You just have to know where and what to look for.

Crack!

"Bad Boys, Bad Boys, watcha gonna do, Whatcha gonna do when they come for you?" Time was, you couldn't tell. I was only twelve or thirteen, but I just couldn't tell. All those mixed up hormones. And that crazy fascination with bikers - bad boy, bikes, boots, and cut off jean jackets. My brother and I used to cut off the sleeves of my Dad's work shirts and use a black marker to design our own colors, then race around the yard on bicycles pretending to be tough bad boys. We were puppies wrestling like big dogs. Practicing puberty. We would spend most of that summer between being tough and stealing my Dad's Penthouse

97

magazines. Of course, we didn't know at that age that ninety-nine percent of those stories were masturbation fiction. I was torn between wanting what the men did to those girls and wishing I was one of those girls.

I used to sit in the window of my bedroom in that big ranch house and dream of cities. I was an angry, sullen boy wishing that I was old enough to leave all the boredom. Angry at what? I did not know. I was unaware that the turbulent emotions were part of the puberty process.

At a time when I should have been interested in horses, the ranch, and male things, I was suddenly interested in fashion, and music, especially the Rolling Stones. Then the world seemed to change overnight. Kennedy, Stonewall, and Prime Minister Treadeau who changed the laws in Canada making homosexuality legal. "The Government has no business in the bedroom of it's citizens," he stated. That was it. Just that word, 'homosexual' triggered and put into place all of the emotions that I had fought with. Strangely enough, what solidified my direction was not the world view, but my father's vehement reactions toward world affairs. I was a REBEL and I couldn't even tell anyone. But just knowing that I was not alone set the stage forever. It may not have changed much outwardly, but it set into motion a series of unconscious decisions that would effect the rest of my life.

Oh, there were still peer pressures to deal with and some wrong turns on that road called life, but the impact was immeasurable. I was able to decipher the differences between need and what would substitute or satisfy my wants. And so this rebel met his match, or rather an equalizer to the needs, fears, and wants of youth. An authoritative figure entered my life at a time when the needs were the greatest, not to mention the most vulnerable: a cop. More accurately, a Royal Canadian Mounted Policeman. I didn't know he was a cop, I was just attracted to all the exuded masculinity. The handcuffs were my favorite.

His guilt matched my own. I found out later that he had more to lose than me. He was off duty when we met and out of uniform, and I was still under age. Unknown to me, he was being transferred so that probably made the approach easier on his part, knowing that it could not last. It was a most exciting time. We had both crossed a line that could not be removed. The fear I encountered upon discovering that he was a policeman matched the excitement that was created because of that fear. It stirred up the raw, sexual, unrelenting desires only youth can provide. Bad boy, rebel with a uniform. This was my first taste of respect on a play level and the beginning of an education in Leather.

Crack!

I had first spotted him in the vendor's area, full of bravado, purchasing a signal whip. The vendor introduced me into the conversation and the topic naturally turned to his experience. I don't remember anything of the conversation except that he made a point of declaring his sexuality as straight and I suppose he just wanted to clarify that kink was all we had in common. He was expecting to use the newly purchased whip at the dungeon party that evening. I shook my head. I couldn't believe it. No practice. No warm-up. Unbelievable.

He was trying hard to be Master of his universe, but his body language screamed the word 'bottom'. His eyes were restless, unsure and his stance insecure, reluctant, and needy. Don't interpret that as relevant to all bottoms, it was just his body language interfering with his perceived needs. It was his suggestion, not mine, that he bottom to my whip. He wanted to, "Just to see what if feels like". After all, he thought he should know what it was that he was subjecting his bottoms to. Yeah, right.

"Okay. Meet me at the Dungeon party later," I told him.

I passed off the conversation, never giving it a second thought. But now, there he stood.

His approach, although unsure, had been respectful and, at least there was honesty in the request.

"Sir, we talked earlier of a curiosity, Sir."

"Are you sure?" I questioned.

"Sir, I would appreciate a sampling of your art…uh, Sir."

He was nervous. No Macho bravado now.

I put my hand on his shoulder, reassuringly, "Just a couple…an introduction."

He nodded sharply.

With little pressure on his shoulder, I turned him toward the wall, leaning him into it and ran my hand down his back. He shivered; out of fear or anticipation of the unknown, I could not tell.

"Remove your shirt and drape it around you neck, like you would a towel."

He obeyed.

"Then place your hands about a shoulder width apart on the wall. I will tell you what I am about to do."

I don't remember where I picked up that little trick about wrapping something around the neck. The T-shirt was security of sorts against a misthrow. It also, unknowingly, placed a sense of insulated comfort with the bottom.

I stood back from the wall and removed my vest. Then I rolled my T-shirt like you would a wet towel and snapped it against his back. It did not strike him, but I swear he jumped like lightning had touched him.

I took a few paces to my toy-bag and collected both my signal whip which I draped around my shoulders, and my coiled galley whip which rested in my left hand. I looked at him again. One jangled bundle of nerves, this one. Turning, I motioned to the submissive that had accompanied me for the evening.

"Stand between him and the wall, provide some support, some physical contact."

She nodded, she understood. Yes, I said SHE - all who share a passion for my whips gain my respect; there are so few that can 'go the distance' with a singletail scene that I admire all of those who wish to experience my chosen craft. This was not the first time, as a senior bottom, she had lent support to a novice. Just that calming effect of another being breathing in your ear can provide solace against that storm known as fear.

I started a slow wash across his back with my T-shirt, just a warm-up. Then, without missing a stroke, I switched to the multi-tailed galley whip. This is a braided whip roughly three feet long, with eight-inch falls attached to the working end. It provides a gentle wash, similar to a flogger, but handles very much like a signal whip for accuracy. It also allows for a smooth build-up and can be deliciously wicked with a little wrist speed. His back was hardening well, and I told him so.

"You are doing well. Relax. Breathe. Let it go."

I am not sure he knew what I meant, but the sound of my voice must have been reassuring because his shoulders dropped a lit tle. The muscles released some of their tension.

"Good, now I am going to change whips," I said, again, not breaking the motion, not missing a stroke as I gently flicked his back with a signal whip. Build it - stop and caress, then build into it some more.

"You are going to hear the whip pop but I am not going to touch you. Wait for it."

I took a half step back and raised my left forefinger to signal the oncoming crack. The young woman providing support blinked acknowledgment over his shoulder, then lowered her face into the wrapped T-shirt. Safety from a miscalculation. Damaging his shoulder with an over-throw is bad form at the least, but to endanger his neck, facial area, or the eyes is unforgivable. That is strictly a no-contact area. The whip split the air at the speed of sound and the sound was thunderous. The second crack, no contact. A third, no contact. The fourth connected like lightning and a four inch red welt appeared on his shoulder. A kiss of the whip.

The whip split the air, connecting.

"Jesus," he hissed through clenched teeth.

I rephrased that for him, *"That's Jesus, Sir."*

"Yes, Sir. Jesus Christ, Sir."

I cracked the whip again just above the skin of his back. The visual was powerful. His back spoke volumes - of fear, not need or understanding.

The visual was powerful. The whip danced above his back.

Do I chance another? I had promised him a couple of strokes. A sampling. The terror was exciting. I slowly arced the whip. No sound emerged, just the feel of the wind across his back. He went rigid with fear and anticipation.

"Relax," I said increasing the arc, "We'll build to another."

I reflected back to the workshop that I had given that afternoon. Being right-handed, I was explaining the use of my left as a guide, a balance and a gun-sight all in one. The ability to put a full arm of force behind the whip while balancing the throw with my left. I compared the similarities to archery; using the full shoulder muscle rather than just the biceps to cock the shot. An interpretation of a complete range of motion. Just try throwing anything with one arm stuck to your side. It is never effective, not to mention inaccurate.

My left arm floated effortlessly in front of me as the whip arm delivered those little popping sounds like foreplay. I raised my left forefinger again, signaling yet another strike. Crack! A matching red welt traced the opposite shoulder.

He dropped like a stone to one knee, hissing through his teeth. Not even able to form words this time. I felt a tightness grip my loins. This was unfair. This was supposed to be a demonstration but it was working for me, too.

The submissive providing support gripped him by the armpits and yanked him back to his feet. His thighs were quivering so hard his jeans were flapping. His eyes were hard.

"Take it," she whispered, "Learn to use it and go with it."

It was beyond his comprehension and he had already had enough.

I dropped the whip into my left hand, reached out and caressed his back between the welts.

"Now you have some idea what you have purchased. What you have in your control."

Sweat flowed freely from his forehead and armpits.

"Come sit," I said, my voice even supportive, "relax while I clean

your back and my whip."

As I guided him back to his seat, I turned and nodded to the woman who had provided support.

"You're up next."

Our needs were to be filled. I had a feeling that mine were more carnal, not that I was aroused.

"Yes, Sir", was all she said, slowly stripping off her shirt, and a shallow smile played across her lips.

I stood in front of him, watching his breathing return to normal. The experience made me cognizant of the reality and intensity I had experienced with my first encounter. It also reminded me of why I came to the community in the first place. Obvious needs were fed in those early days. I was aware of the hunger, the vulnerability, and the exposure to an inner self that had purposely been avoided. My mind went over the tender, unwanted memories that I knew I would have to face and conquer eventually. But I never expected to find the answers in a world of Leather and SM. The Leather lifestyle was supposed to provide lustful and physical satisfactions, not emotional answers. I also never realized how deeply some of my hurts were buried. The answers have become more difficult to define as my experiences grow, with the definitions becoming increasingly broad.

Ask me what Leather is now and I would probably stare at you with an incredibly baffled look. Given some time, I could probably formulate and articulate a reasonable answer to such a broad question, but parables seem to work better as definitions through comparisons. Draw your own conclusions.

After it was cleaned, I coiled the signal whip over the back of the chair where the novice sat nursing his welts. Gathering my toy bag, I sorted through several items. I could have sworn there had been a blindfold in there. I glanced over in the direction of the woman waiting against the wall. Had she read my mind? There she stood, naked from the waist up, facing the wall, wearing it. This was promising to be a great weekend.

What is Leather? I suppose that, if you think you are, then you are.

Visual manifestations aside, whatever your perception of the term, if it fits - then proudly wear it. Any interpretation of the meaning will apply to whatever you decide it should represent. Two things need to happen here. Your interpretation must suit you and not have been borrowed or applied to your Leather-self (by someone else's definition), and you have to believe in it. The difference shows, whether you are just dressing the part, or whether leather is part of your make-up. Body language says more about who you are than a uniform ever will, including gender identity or preference; your own, that is, not that of whom you wish to sleep with.

I find it interesting that gays and lesbians have been mixing-it-up and playing together within the last decade, yet still retain their individual sexual identities. Add fetish folk, and the full spectrum of sexual identity and leather takes on a very broad scope in which to place yourself. I believe, and I may draw a lot of criticism here, that gays and lesbians are able to play together so successfully because of an inherent understanding of equality. This comment is not intended to denigrate the kinky straight population, just an explanation of my own observations.

Equality manifests itself in reality in that, if two men or two women enter a scene, play, and then close that scene, there are no societal pressures present before or after to change the equality of the players. It is important to remember that this is my reality, based solely on my observations and an upbringing and education fitted to a specific era. Geography and exposure to various other aspects may allow for different conclusions.

Two men going into a scene are still two men when that scene is over, no matter what their chosen life roles are or what their roles are within the scene. To a large degree, gender supplies that equality. I believe the same to be true for lesbian players. So, by extension, a gay man and a lesbian playing together share an equality that is understood because of their individual preferred sexuality. In other words, because they are both gay. Now, I may add confusion to this by saying that a gay man and a straight woman playing together may share that same equality. I have never witnessed that balance between straight men and straight women or, for that matter, a lesbian and a straight man. The scene or play itself may be balanced because of what was negotiated, but the equality of the players before and after that scene is not.

There is the shared belief that Leather, as a costume, is not an end to itself, but rather, something deeper. It is spiritual, but not religious. Most Leatherfolk may not be able to put into words what their Leather means to them on a spiritual level, but it is visible nonetheless. Observe any group of Leatherfolk in any setting and they seem to be shrouded in myth and mystery. That is part of the allure, part of the attraction to the culture; that we may know something that others have not yet discovered. Thus, Leather is mostly self-defining; a visible expression of inner fortitude. It is a concept rather than an application of definitive parameters. This is not to take away from the rigidity of Old Guard morals, but rather to augment their reality. Follow all the rules you want. If you don't believe in where you are as a Leatherman, this is a rather moot point.

Walk the part, but not part of the walk. How do you explain such a concept? How do you substantiate an existence that is so far removed from what most consider normal and yet, is more central to the heart of what all living beings wish to accomplish? That stripping away of layers to reveal what? A rebirth? Again I am alluding to an endless circle of spirituality.

Crack!

Fresh horses. All kinds of images come to mind with those two words. The most obvious being a new start on an endless quest where the smallest things will trigger a new interest or even a new direction. Ever notice how these beginnings are always singular? And they always occur on the last day of your vacation? In other words, the things you were most prepared for, or anticipated, never became reality but, in it's place, a new revelation sparks all kinds of new ideas. Possibly because the things you were so used to, so comfortable with, become so repetitive that they reach a plateau and level you off. This new idea changes your present direction and sometimes, your understanding of everything you think you know.

Have you ever discovered some incredible place to eat? For example, a place that just hit the spot, satisfying a craving you weren't even aware of, on the last day of a holiday? You know you may never be back this way again. The worst part of this discovery is that it becomes a memory that is irreplaceable and impossible to repeat because of the expectations or anticipation placed on it. It becomes a new and refreshing rare treasure.

I try, although I know that I am not always successful, to approach all my experiences with the possibility of that wild card. Even with the parameters outlined and the choreography in place - with basic expectations completed - there is always that chance of something new.

Anthologies.

I don't know why, but I believe in the need to remember what my experiences mean to me. Not that they could, or should, ever be compared to anyone else's experiences, but possibly a pattern of comparisons will help to measure a collective spirit of the community. There is probably not much that I could relate that would ever make a difference in someone's life, but hopefully the things I relate will enable some to say, "Yes, I can relate", or, "That is how I feel. I just never put words to it."

I run the risk here of being just a little off-center compared to the experiences of the vast majority of Leatherfolk. My need to examine even the simplest of experiences is just my way of tackling, or maybe justifying, the quality of those experiences.

As a culture, we seem to have a difficult time explaining how we feel about what it is we do. We pass along our knowledge through a series of initiations or repetitive exposures to those things that mean something to us, relating experiences that have shaped or defined what our culture means to us on an individual basis.

Crack!

I have had my metal tested many times as a Leatherman. It is much like being gay. The needs override what we would some times choose as lifestyles. I think the saying goes, "Those things that do not kill me, make me stronger." I disagree. It is hard to believe in what you do when you are up to your ass in alligators and the original job was to drain the swamp. So take no prisoners and have no regrets. After all, you are the only person that can do the job.

I have lost self-control, to the point of wanting to hit someone out of anger, only once since acknowledging my Leather existence. I felt provoked to the point of frustration with someone who I felt should have known better - a Leatherman with more experience than me. This particular Leatherman walked up to the bottom accompanying me, full collar and lock showing, grabbed him and laid a lengthy kiss on him. I realize that this may not be an unusual thing to do for some members of our community, but this happened in defined Leather-space. Old Guard. I should mention that my boy and his Leatherman had had a previous relationship that ended badly. Apparently, he had disappeared out of the boy's life after several years of contracting - with no warning and no explanation - revealing an obvious lack of respect for someone in his charge.

We were all attending a Meat 'n Greet prior to a Drummer Contest in Seattle. Whether he was trying to impress someone I was unaware of, or just to prove he could still Top the boy, escapes me. Either that or the beer he had been drinking was maneuvering his testosterone.

I tapped him on the shoulder and said, "Excuse me, don't touch what you don't have the key for."

"Fuck off!" was his reply.

The poor boy, eyes as big as saucers, looked in my direction for guidance. It was obvious he understood the awkward position that he had been placed in. I, and the crowd around me, was so shocked by this response to my claim of ownership that the space surrounding him and my bottom quickly evaporated in a circle of disbelief. All eyes turned to me.

I am sure he was secretly pleased that I was angered beyond reason. Before I could react, he just turned and left. We, thankfully, never saw him again that weekend. I still get angry when I think about that event but I have learned that, for all the posturing some Leatherfolk do, there is not a lot of depth within. Those same circumstance today would draw more amusement from me than the deep anger incurred at the time. I think it would reflect on that particular Leatherman's inability to understand his role, rather than my need to be defensive or assertive about mine.

That does not mean that I should not defend my honor or my family, only that he was the one trespassing on private property and should have known better. His inability to look me in the eye since that incident is reward enough for the infraction, since an apology would be never be forthcoming. Not to mention the eyes in the crowd that witnessed and then passed judgment about him as a Leatherman. Ignoring the situation after it had occurred created even more of a stir within the community.

The boy learned, too, that his decisions are honored and treated with respect. He may be a boy out of choice but that does not take away his ability to control a situation that is not to his liking. Nor does the choice to be a boy delineate his position within the *family, or community.*

Crack!

*"Rape is about aggression and lack of power. SM is about equal-
ity and exchange of power." Strange how I have to roll over in
bed in the middle of the night to jot down these little notes. It is
when I wake that everything becomes cloudy with real-life stuff
overlapping my thoughts. And those early hours before sunlight
bring out the most exciting and erotic thoughts also.*

*Envision two men standing side by side in a social setting - both
of similar builds, looks, and dressed in leathers, casually enjoying the evening but one holds a coiled whip in his left hand. That
whip makes a statement at once. The statement being both political and religious. Political in the sense that it sets the two apart,
divided even within the Leather community, and religious in a
spiritual manner, a belief in something structured, if not profound,
to the viewer. Also, depending on the setting, is the whip there
for shock value or advertising? Chances are, if you see some
one carrying or displaying an item of such advertised interest,
then that person knows how to use, apply, and respect that imple-
ment, be it handcuffs, floggers, knives, or teddy bears. The skill
level necessary to master such implements of exquisite pleasure,
(yes…even I can see the humor in teddy bears) takes finesse
that requires more than the strength of Leather visibility. It is a
controlled dark dance. A ballet.*

*The whip requires a level of control that carries itself over to the
whip master. It provides an air of mastery that shines like a bea-
con on one who knows its power; a blinding, flashing, warning
light on those that have not yet mastered subtleties of that control, both at the business end of the whip and in their hearts. And
for those that understand the extremes within their reach, that
skill becomes defined as a visible extension of an inner control
that is as immovable as solid rock. Yet, it has a touch of tenderness that lies invisible just beneath the surface.*

I do not often have the opportunity to review my education or experiences
with much clarity. I mean, it is hard to analyze or decipher when certain
events or turning points become educational revelations. Too often, the
experiences run together without a defining grade system to tell you

where you fit, as is the case in more structured environments. There again, in my interpretation, lies the value of the Old Guard. I keep alluding to this generation of Leathermen, but it is my only measure of reference to which I can relay my thoughts.

The ability of a more experienced Leatherman to pass along knowledge and the respective rewards symbolizes those graduated areas of education. In other words, "earning your Leathers," one piece at a time. And again, as I have said before, age plays a very small role within the learning curve. The older, dominant 'Daddy' figure is not only common to the culture in terms of knowledge, but is also a very powerful erotic symbol within the framework of our established families. Families by choice, not birthright. Usually, the learning curve and the analogies that accompany it, is only visible by passing along your knowledge to the people interested in entering the community.

You realize you are a 'Daddy' when you have the ability to articulate and decipher answers to questions in relationship to your own passage through the trials and errors of education. Like learning to drive a car with a blindfold on, bumping into all kinds of things before settling into a comfort zone from which to sit still and explore the available information. I still enjoy the naive freshness and shy honesty accompanying the questions and it is especially gratifying to watch the 'lights go on' when trying to explain monogamy, especially after a beer or two in social settings. There seems to be some sinister need to see couples fail or to split them apart. Almost a justification of the torn and ragged lives some Leatherfolk lead. Just as most people like to see large corporations fail or pubic figures in high places exposed, there is always this morbid fascination of failure. And yet, success stories in our culture shine above the failures, validating a culture that both destroys and praises itself.

Crack!

A highway of life littered with tragedy. And yet, the only real education.

Mike. He was interesting to watch. It was also fearful to watch him because he had not learned to parcel out his feelings. He didn't know how to tap into them and let them dissipate or escalate into useful tools within the scene. He didn't realize that doors could be opened just enough for a glimpse of the need waiting inside. It seemed he would approach the door and open it just a crack during every scene, but the flood of emotions behind it could not be contained so simply. Possibly, it was all too over whelming and all that emotional baggage just cascaded out; like standing behind a dump truck and teasing the tailgate with a flogger, accidentally hitting the latch and dumping everything on the same unsuspecting Top. Possibly, no one had taken the time to teach him how to allocate those feelings or more likely, he had rushed through the early states of his Leather and pushed limits that were not yet understood.

*I watched with a sort of fascinated horror at his brave attempts to peer into the plate-glass windows of a culture that reduced his existence to one of looking through keyholes, wondering why he wasn't seeing the whole picture. He wanted so badly to be part of it all and know it all....yesterday. It was all so exciting, so erotic and lustful, that he needed to throw himself into it feet-first and damn the torpedoes. There was no time for building bridges, paying your dues, or asking directions. It reminds me of a T-shirt emblazoned with, "**JUST DO ME**." He was **READY**, capital letters, cum-fuck-me-**R-E-A-D-Y**. But for what? Anything, anywhere, **JUST DO ME**. Sensory overload. It would have been almost comical if it wasn't so tragic at the same time. It was like watching a puppy grow through those awkward stages of tripping over it's own limbs.*

I grew up in a small town where the hardware store was literally the department store. It was a masculine place, and they sold everything, from nuts and bolts, to guns. I also remember being quite fearful of the look that would show up on the men's faces when they picked up a gun. How that look would grow and change across their faces, as if by some trick or osmosis there was a power relinquished from the gun to the bearer. It was a dangerous look, if only for an instant. That "I'm ready" look, that Just-point-me-in-the-right-direction, if-it-moves-I'll-kill-it look. Such incredible power held in their hands.

Some would replace the gun on the counter with shaky hands, fearful, or maybe respectful of that power. Others would caress the gun before replacing it and then rub their sweaty hands on their thighs, intoxicated with their own fantasies of wielding such power.

We all know men and women who abuse power in many forms. Most are not even aware of the infractions because they are so ingrained or deeply rooted. They appear normal to their personal makeup. Like rust, it is a slowly eroding sense of self-esteem, festering under a veil of abuse toward oneself or fired blindly at whomever passes near.

What program provides just the right amount of support to allow for the exploration of personal fantasies and/or tragedies? Where do you jump on that carousel of Leather events, workshops, clubs, dungeon parties, ad nauseam? With so much information available, it would be easy to get caught up in the fantasy version of the community. And why not? The sex is hot and fun and constant. But it is also lonely, and the only way to battle loneliness is with another trick, another flogging, or another orgasm. Just one of the many reasons that there are established families within our loose-knit community. So when you get tired of tricking, approach one of the community leaders and ask, sincerely, for direction.

There are non-visible community members who are always in the background, but are the backbone community. They may rarely go to the bar or attend social events but they have always been there for support and answers within the core structure of communities. Call them leaders, mentors, Daddy's, or even Old Guard, but call them. A word of caution, *you may not like some of the answers to your questions*. You also may not be asking the *right* questions, but at least the answers will be honest and so will the direction. You may have to try several times to find the answers that fit your particular situation, but do not give up. Curt or evasive inquiries about your interest may only be the result of a protective system. Sort of a self-defense mechanism, reactive to the prying and the curious. Be prepared for it. It will happen. Besides, if the need is really there, you will find ways of making contact on more than a sexual level.

Where should I take you from here? A self-defining journey of experiences that can only be explained through the storytelling process. Those experiences cannot be repeated but they can be re-created in most forms to help explore the variety of emotions involved. In fact, I spend a lot of time trying to re-create some of my favorite fantasies and the physical rewards that accompanied them. That is like saying that there are no poor orgasms; there are good ones and there are great ones. Take some time for yourself; you have a lot to give someone. Remember I said watch the eyes? The eyes are the mirror to the soul and, if the eyes are dull, maybe the polish on the mirror could use some attention. If someone is unhappy with their life, the eyes are the first place to search for clues. So much is masked or hidden behind that thin veil of those eyes.

This is not about ego. That should be checked at the door. It is about facing unknowns and the chance to escape, without explanation, into a world that needs no justification to anyone. It seems to me that only those who have faced great pain or personal crisis within their lives really get the significance of the message. That message comes in many forms, of which Leather is just one. Compared to a pie, if only one slice is our commitment to Leather, the pie is not complete without that one slice, but the rest of the pie also supports that single slice. Art imitates life or life imitates art.

There seems to be an extension to the equation where understanding becomes inherent to the lifestyle; rather than Leather being a room that can be slipped into, or out of, at will when the need arises or subsides. Rather, it comes an invisible extension of our personalities. It is nothing that can be distinguished in any uniform way because it is unique to the bearer. Possibly, you have guessed by now that this whole Leather thing has very little to do with Leather as defined within erotic parameters, and lots to do with life in more general terms. That may be pretty broad, but when something so profound effects so much of everyday life, it becomes very much a part of existence. It is soul and it is spiritual.

In Leather, Don.

Other titles from Daedalus Publishing Company:

The Master's Manual $15.95
A Handbook of Erotic Dominance
In this book, author Jack Rinella examines various aspects of erotic dominance, including SM, safety, sex, erotic power, techniques and more.

SlaveCraft $15.95
Roadmaps for Erotic Servitude
principles, skills and tools
Guy Baldwin, author of Ties That Bind, joins forces with a grateful slave to produce this gripping and personal account on the subject of consensual slavery.

The Compleat Slave $15.95
Creating and Living an Erotic Dominant/submissive Lifestyle
In this highly anticipated follow-up to The Master's Manual, author Jack Rinella continues his in-depth exploration of Dominant/submissive relationships.

Learning the Ropes $12.95
A Basic Guide to Fun S/M Lovemaking
This book, by S/M expert Race Bannon, guides the reader through the basics of safe and fun S/M.

My Private Life $14.95
Real Experiences of a Dominant Woman
Within these pages, the author, Mistress Nan, allows the reader a brief glimpse into the true private life of an erotically dominant woman.

Leathersex $16.95
A Guide for the Curious Outsider and the Serious Player
Written by renound S/M author Joseph Bean, the reader will find much wisdom within this volume about this often misunderstood form of erotic expression

Consensual Sadomasochism $16.95
How To Talk About It And How To Do It Safely
Authors William A. Henkin, Ph. D. and Sybil Holiday, CCSSE combine their knowledge and expertise in this unique examination of erotic consensual sado masochism.

Beneath The Skins $12.95
The New Spirit And Politics Of The Kink Community
This book by Ivo Dominguez, Jr. examines the many issues facing the modern leather/SM/fetish community.

Ties That Bind $16.95
The SM/Leather/Fetish Erotic Style
Issues, Commentaries and Advice
The early writings of well-known psychotherapist and respected member of the leather community Guy Baldwin have been compiled to create this SM classic

Leathersex Q&A $16.95
Questions About Leathersex and the Leather Lifestyle Answered
In this interesting and informative book, author Joseph Bean answers a wide variety of questions about leathersex sexuality.

Leather and Latex Care $10.95
How To Keep Your Leather And Latex Looking Great
This concise book by Kelly J. Thibault gives the reader all they need to know to keep their leather and latex items looking great

Between The Cracks $18.95
The Daedalus Anthology of Kinky Verse
Editor Gavin Dillard has compiled this impressive selection of poetry from well-known authors that celebrates the edgier side of sexuality.

The Leather Contest Guide $12.95
A Handbook For Promoters, Contestants, Judges and Titleholders
International Mr. Leather and Mr. National Leather Association contest winner Guy Baldwin is the author of this truly complete guide to the leather contest

Ordering Information

Orders may be placed over the phone at:

323.666.2121

Orders may also be placed via email at:

order@DaedalusPublishing.com

To order any Daedalus titles by mail, send your name, mailing address, and the names of the books you would like to purchase, along with a check or money order made payable to "Daedalus Publishing Company". Do not send cash. Send to:

Daedalus Publishing Company
2140 Hyperion Ave
Los Angeles, CA 90027

California residents should add 8.25% sales tax. All orders should include a $4.25 shipping charge for the first book, plus $1.00 for each additional book added to the total of the order.

Since many of our publications deal with sexuality issues, please include a signed statement that you are at least 21 years of age with any order.

Please visit our website at:

http://www.daedaluspublishing.com